Secrets of the Bikini Competitor

Everything you need to rock the stage and win your competition

By Valerie Wiest

Secrets of the Bikini Competitor

Valerie Wiest

Author

Valerie Wiest

Editor

Valerie Wiest

First Published 2015

This book may be purchased for educational, business, or sales promotional use. Online edition is also available for this title. For more

Secrets of the Bikini Competitor

Valerie Wiest

information, contact our corporate/institutional sales department:
www.valeriewiest.com/contact

Contents

My Story

Hi! Thanks so much for getting my book. I am excited for you to start your journey! I wanted to write this book to clear up some of the confusion about bikini competitions and to help competitors succeed without falling into unhealthy habits.

I entered my first competition in 2010. It was just after I had gotten married and I was going through a tough time maintaining my independence and self in my relationship with my husband. Since I loved working out but never had a goal in mind for my workouts, I thought training for a fitness competition would be a great idea.

In 2010 bikini was a brand new division and I did not even know it existed so I searched online for a figure competition and entered one about 2 hours away from my home. I did everything on a shoestring budget. I made my own training and diet plans based on things I had read online. I chose my music, practiced the mandatory poses for a few hours and bought a cut-rate suit.

I went in clueless about the industry and my results showed my lack of knowledge—I placed last in both divisions that I entered. Even though my placings weren't where I wanted them to be, I still had a great time. The girls I met were super nice and I felt proud of myself for putting myself out there and following through on a goal.

Years passed and I became a mom, I also became a personal trainer and a Pilates instructor. I started reading fitness magazines and following fitness blogs and I learned about the bikini division. It had always been my dream to prove to other moms that having kids didn't have to be an excuse keeping you from achieving the body of your dreams. I started to get the itch to do another fitness competition. This time I chose to compete in bikini, since I felt my frame was better suited for it.

Valerie Wiest

Determined to do better than my last show, I hired a coach: IFBB Pro Jessica Jessie, who has been invaluable to my journey. Jessica taught me what the judges were looking for, how to train, what to eat and how to pose. Turns out, I should have been practicing posing every day, not just a few hours before the show!

My goal for my first bikini competition was to look like I belonged on stage and to place higher than last place. I ended up placing second in my first show! I was over the moon! Since then, I have placed top 3 in all of the local shows I have competed in and top 15 in the national level show I attended.

I wanted to share what I have learned with you so that you too can train smarter, not harder and learn the secrets of getting in the best shape of your life!

Typos:

In order to keep this book affordable, it is self-edited. Yes, I am one of those people who knows the difference between "their, there, and they're" and it totally annoys me when I see them used in the wrong way. But sometimes, even us self-proclaimed "grammar Nazis" miss something. If you find a typo, misspelling or mistake send a quick e-mail to Valerie@valeriewiest.com with the location and mistake and I'll be sure to edit it. If you do, I'll be forever grateful!

Free Bonuses

For a limited time, you can get my meal prep guide for free. Just go to www.bikinimealprep.com to download it.

Join our private Bikini Competitor Facebook Group at facebook.com/groups/bikinicompetitor. Let's help each other achieve success by sharing tips, strategies and questions. Enjoy the rest of the book!

Valerie Wiest

So You Want To Be a Bikini Competitor

What does competing take?

Want to be a bikini competitor? Think bikini competitions are all about looking hot and prancing around on stage? Well, I'm here to tell you that it is not all glamorous. Competing is tough and takes a lot out of you. You will be pushing yourself in your workouts while tapering down the amount of food you eat. As if the physical effects of the training were not enough, the mental anxiety and stress of trying to lose weight and get ready for your competition will also take a toll on you.

Here is straight talk on what it takes to compete. I say this not to discourage you, but to give you realistic expectations and help you to prepare for what is ahead.

First, is the commitment of time. You need time for meal prep, working out and posing practice. For me, meal prep takes about 1 hour at the start of the week and then 15 min. each day in preparing my food for the day. For workouts you will want to clock in about 1.5-2 hours per day. Let's say approximately 30+ minutes of cardio per day and 1+ hours of weight training. We will discuss training later in the Bikini Prep Workout Plan section. If you have time in your schedule for this, then you are well on your way! Training and dieting are about 50% of the battle.

The next thing you should be prepared for is the cost of competing. Competing isn't cheap! I spent well over $1000 on my first competition. And while this book is full of tips on how you can save money while competing, registration for most NPC shows is around $100 and the NPC card (required to compete) is $125 so that is $225 just to step on stage. If you are struggling with money right now, it is probably NOT the time to compete.

Discipline is another factor that will come into play. Please keep in mind that a competition diet is not your standard diet and exercise plan and may not be appropriate for everyone. You must have enough discipline to stay focused and committed to the diet and exercise plan or you will not have a chance at winning. If you are going to put 50% into competing, please expect that there will be some girls giving it 110% and if you cannot find the place in your life for that kind of dedication and discipline this may not be for you.

Finally, I recommend that you be in a stable happy place when you compete. The decrease in food alone will affect your body's hormones, which may mess with your moods and emotions. Basically, competing has the potential to wreak havoc on your emotional state and if you are already in a bad place, you become even more vulnerable. Trust me, I have experienced this and have talked to others who have as well. Remember, this is a hobby it should be fun, not something that destroys your life.

These guidelines are designed to help you decide if entering a bikini competition is right for you. Competing is not for everyone. If you are not in a good place to compete right now, don't worry, you can always come back to competitions later in your life. But be honest with yourself, entering a bikini competition is not a good reason to destroy yourself physically, emotionally and financially.

What is your goal and why?

Still interested in competing? Good, I was hoping I didn't lose you in that last section! Before you get started, I recommend that you take a look at what you are looking to get out of this experience. That means establishing a goal. Setting clear goals and finding a purpose in competing will keep you motivated as things get challenging.

Your goal for competing should be a compelling one that will help you push past difficulties that you may face. It should be something that resonates with you: Do you want to compete to celebrate transforming your body? Are you looking to inspire other moms to live a fit and healthy life? Are you trying to create a career in the fitness industry?

Once you have recognized your goal, ask yourself why you chose that goal. For example, if your goal is to get your pro card—why? Will it help you achieve what you want? Make sure your goal is about you, not what others think of you. Your goal should be serving some purpose in your life. This will help you to maintain a strong sense of motivation.

For example, my goal was to demonstrate to other new moms and to myself that having a baby doesn't mean that you can't also have a body you love. I also wanted to make a name for myself in the fitness industry. I felt like competing would give me the experience and knowledge to help others achieve similar results.

Write your goal(s) down and put them somewhere so that you can see them when you are having a rough time. They must be powerful enough to keep you going even when the going gets tough!

So You Want to Go "Pro"

For many people going "pro" or earning their pro card is their main goal in competing. To go pro, you must compete and be one of the top competitors in a local show designated as a national qualifier (usually top 3 or top 5 qualify). Then, you must compete and win in your class at a national level show. Sometimes the top two winners in the class at a national show both earn their pro cards. You can find out more about how to win pro status at each national show here: http://npcnewsonline.com/rules/.

Once you earn your pro card you can compete in pro shows and earn money as you win. Many want to earn their pro card to gain recognition in the fitness industry and hopefully gain sponsorship, which I will talk about later on. If that is your goal, good for you! Just know that earning your pro card does not necessarily mean that either of these things will happen. In fact, in the NPC you must pay a yearly fee to maintain your "pro" status and you give up your rights to compete in any other organization as long as you hold that title.

14

Organizations

Once you have settled on a goal and decided that you are ready to enter your competition, you will want to consider which organization you would like to register with. Some organizations are "not tested," which means many of the competitors may be using banned substances to help them achieve their desired look (yes, even in the bikini division). Others are tested (usually with a lie detector test issued by a police officer). If you are considering competing in a natural organization, you will want to make sure you know what substances are considered "banned." There are many organizations to choose from and I have broken down a list of the most popular amateur organizations below:

- NPC: An untested organization started by Joe and Ben Weider. This is, in my opinion, the most popular and prestigious organization. However, politics and drugs can play a role into how well you do. Pro level is IFBB (International Federation of Body Building)
- OCB: A tested organization. The bikini division has a bigger production with a T-walk and song selection. Pro Level is IFPA
- NANBF: The North American Natural Bodybuilding Federation was founded with a goal to promote drug tested body building shows.
- WBFF: The WBFF was created by an athlete, for the athletes. It features pro and amateur bodybuilding, male/female fitness model/male muscle model, and women's figure.
- NGA: Drug tested, non-profit organization
- INBF: Natural organization with bikini division.
- UNBA: The United Natural Bodybuilding Association is a natural and drug tested organization.

The training in this book will focus mostly on competing in the NPC because that is the organization in which I have competed the most. However, because the standards are similar, much of the information provided in this book will help in other organizations.

Choosing a show

Ok, so you have decided you are ready to compete! Congratulations! Now you need to choose your show. Once you have decided the organization in which you would like to compete, you can go on their website and find a list of upcoming competitions. You can search NPC bikini competitions here: http://npcnewsonline.com/schedules/

The first thing you will want to consider, when picking a show, is when you will realistically be physically ready to compete. While there is no exact science to this, most bikini girls are between 8-12% body fat with a solid base of muscle. I will talk in more details about what is required for the "bikini look" later in the book. However, you should know that building a base of muscle will take longer than losing body fat. If you are starting out as a beginner lifter, I would recommend taking at least a year to build up a good base of muscle for competing.

If you already have a good base of muscle and just need to slim down a bit or make minor tweaks to your physique, a good place to start is finding your body fat percentage. There are many ways to do this including special scales, calipers, and the BOD POD®. Although some systems used to measure body fat are more effective than others, the most important thing to keep in mind is that you should be consistent with the time of day and with the person who takes your measurements. For example, having your coach take measurements\ every Saturday at 9:00am would be a good idea. By comparing your measurements to those taken under similar conditions, you reduce your chances for error. Tracking your progress numerically will help you stay accountable to your goal and help you quantify your progress. Once you find your body fat and measurements you have a baseline for the rest of your training.

The maximum percentage of body fat you can lose in a week is 1%. (Earle, 2008) Thus, the number of percentage points you would like to drop your body fat level is the minimum number of weeks you will need to train for your competition. For example, if you are 20% body fat and you want to reach 8-12% body fat, give yourself at least 12 weeks to lean down. It is best to be conservative in the amount of time you allow for fat loss to account for plateaus or setbacks.

Another great way to track progress and assess your body is to take body measurements. You can find your body measurements with a tape measure. I recommend at least measuring your neck, upper arm, bust, waist, hips, upper thigh and calf once a week to track changes in your body. Just like you did with your body fat measurements, it is best if you can take your physical measurements under approximately the same conditions each week. This offers you another way to objectively track your progress and ensure that you are headed in the right direction. In bikini we are looking for hourglass proportions and a waist to hip ratio of about 0.66. That is the classic 36-24-36 ratio.

You can also use subjective measurements to assess your current look and track your progress. I think one of the best ways to do this is to take pictures of yourself in a bikini in your front and back pose. Not only is this a great way to see the changes in your body through the process, but you can also compare those pictures to photos of the bikini division pro's front and back pose. This will give you an idea of how your body looks compared to the best in the industry. It will also help you determine your weak points and analyze what areas you need to bring up and what areas you need to bring down.

Using this data, you will be able to determine how far out to schedule your show. As I mentioned before, you may even want to give yourself a few extra weeks to ensure that everything goes smoothly.

Valerie Wiest

Once you have decided approximately when you would like to compete, you should narrow down the location. I HIGHLY recommend starting with a show close to your home. As I mentioned before, this is a very expensive sport and if you can save costs by staying close to home, do it! In addition, don't under estimate the convenience of being close to home if you forget something or need something last minute. Also, being in familiar surroundings will reduce your stress and help you to stay in your comfort zone before the big event.

One other consideration to make before you choose a show is the size of the show and whether or not it is a "national qualifier." Placing top 5 or top 3 (depending on the show) in a national qualifier allows you to compete at the national level. If you are planning to go for your pro card this is a necessary step. If that is your goal, I would recommend competing in a National Qualifier for your first show if you are able to. You may also want to find out who is judging the shows if you plan on going for your pro card. The more exposure you can get to national and pro level judges the more you will be recognized and thus, you will more likely be recognized you advance in the levels. This can work to your favor if you continue to improve your physique and demonstrate good sportsmanship. In the NPC there are a few big shows that are known for having top judges and winning at these shows helps set you up for a win at the national level.

Once you have decided on the show you would like to attend you need to sign up. Even if the competition is weeks away I recommend signing up as soon as possible. First of all, many competitions charge a late registration fee if you register after a certain date, and since this late fee can be pretty expensive, you'll want to make sure you register on time! Additionally, I find that it is easier to back out if you wait to register. By registering early, you cement the idea and date of the competition in your head and will be more likely to follow through on your goals.

For NPC shows, you can find the schedules at http://npcnewsonline.com/schedules/. Once you are on the site, select the show you are interested in and it will take you to the promoter's website. There, you will be able to print out the application or fill it out online if that option is available. If you fill the application out online there is usually an option to make payment online too. If you choose to mail it in, most applications require that you send a money order for your application fee (you can get that at the post office). You will also need an NPC card active for the year in which you compete. These can usually be purchased on the day of the show at check in (make sure you bring cash) and they are also now available for purchase online at http://npcnewsonline.com/join-the-npc/. A word about NPC cards—they are only good for the year in which they were purchased, NOT for a year from the purchase date (i.e. if you buy your card in November 2017, it will expire December 31, 2017.)

That pretty much sums up the registration process. Once you are registered get ready, the fun is about to begin!

Hiring a Coach

Now that you are registered for your competition you will want to decide if you will use a coach. Initially, I flip flopped on my decision to hire a coach mostly because as a certified personal trainer and avid fitness researcher (technical term for someone who spends way too much time on the internet looking at fitness blogs/articles/forums), I felt like everything I needed to know, I knew already or I could find online. Boy was I wrong.

My coach blew my mind after our first training session. I had been following a traditional bodybuilding plan- heavy compound lifts with small amounts of cardio and lots of ab work. My coach explained what the judges were looking for. Whereas I thought they were just looking for a fit body, she explained that great glutes are the focus of judging in bikini. She showed me a ton of glute exercises that I had never done before and had me incorporate plyometrics to help me build my booty. She changed up my cardio, to help sculpt my glutes and she told me that all the ab work I was doing had to go. Turns out that the tons of oblique crunches and twists I was doing were actually making my waist BIGGER! Yikes! (I am already shaped kind of like a ruler so I need to do anything I can to narrow my waist and create curves). Basically, she transformed my entire exercise program and gave me the knowledge I needed to succeed.

After a week or two of working with my trainer, I started noticing huge changes in my glutes, waist and shoulders. My body was becoming the hourglass shape that I wanted. It also simplified things because each week she gave me a plan so all I had to do was what was written down for me. It took the guess work out of training and dieting.

Besides training, my coach taught me exactly what to expect. Because of her experience, she was able to help me with jewelry, hair, make-up and choosing the right suit. She even gave me a plan to follow for the week up to the competition to prepare my skin and come in looking my absolute best. If I ever had a moment of panic, she was there to calm me down and help find a solution. In addition, she kept me accountable, checking in with me once a week to make sure the plan was going well.

In my first competition (when I did not use a coach), I had barely practiced posing and I had no idea that it played such a big role in the competition results. This time, the main thing my coach worked on with me was posing. She helped me streamline a routine that showed off my physique in the best possible way.

Finally, my coach helped me make connections. Because she was a past competitor, she knew the judges and introduced me to a ton of people so I didn't feel awkward and alone back stage. Not only did it help me build new relationships, but it gave me confidence, which I think showed on stage.

Choosing a coach is totally up to you but I highly recommend finding a qualified coach. How do you know if the coach is qualified? They should be a certified personal trainer and nutritionist. They should also have experience preparing other girls for bikini competitions. You can also ask for references to see how their clients have done and what their clients have to say about them.

However, having a qualified coach is not enough in itself. Make sure your coach matches your personality and training philosophy. If you are very sensitive, don't choose a tough love coach! Similarly, if you can't see yourself doing hours of cardio each day, don't choose a coach who requires that of you. Not everyone will work well with every coach and that is ok! Find someone that you have a connection with because you will need to trust them throughout this process.

You can find more information about my coach Jessica Jessie on her website at www.JessicaJessie.com

Online vs. Local Coach

In my opinion, a qualified local coach is always a better choice. A local coach will be more available and will be better able to tweak your diet, training and posing plan as necessary. There is so much you can learn and gain from someone being in person that is missing in Skype chats or internet conversations. Not to mention what you will gain from what a local coach knows about the local fitness industry. While an online coach is an ok option if you don't have any qualified local coaches available to you, I highly recommend seeking out a local coach if one is available.

Choosing a suit

Once you have set your competition date and decided whether or not to use a coach, you will want to choose a bikini. Bikinis typically take a few weeks to process so make sure you order as soon as possible once you know your show date.

Choosing a competition bikini can be confusing when you are just getting started because the choices can be overwhelming. It is hard to know what the judges are looking for if you are unfamiliar with bikini competitions.

First, let's start with where to buy your suit. All of the suits I have worn have been from Waterbabies and I have been super happy with their products. If you are interested in checking out other designers, here is a list of some popular suit makers:

Waterbabies: https://www.waterbabiesbikini.com/
Suits You: http://www.suitsyouswimwear.com/
Ravish Sands: http://www.ravishsands.com/
CJ's Elite: http://cynthia-james.com/
Lydia Conti: http://www.lidiaconti.com/

Color

Next let's talk about color. You want to choose a bold, dark color that will not get washed out on stage. Primary colors tend to pop so start by looking at blues, reds and yellows. Besides primary colors bold purple and green can look great too. Orange and pink tend to blend in with the spray tan and pink can come off as cliché. Do not choose pastels or white. These colors tend to wash out under the bright lights and it is easy for the spray tan to rub off on lighter colors making the suit look dirty. I also don't recommend going crazy with patterns or lace that could distract from your physique. If you know you look good in a certain color, choose that one!

Fit

There will be lots of options for fit. For smaller busted girls, definitely go with a molded cup and ask for pockets so that you can stuff your top. Usually, you can choose the size and shape of the top and bottoms. For the top, I find that it is best to stick with the traditional triangle top rather than selecting something different or asymmetrical. You may have the option to choose between skinny or regular triangle based on your bust size. Larger bust sizes will want the regular triangle, while smaller busted girls can opt for the skinny triangle top. For bottoms, make sure the back is a scrunch to enhance the roundness of your rear. For NPC, the guideline for suits is that they should be in good taste but, keeping this guideline in mind, less coverage shows off more of your hard work! If you have any questions about fit and sizing reach out to the suit company and ask before you buy. Most of the bikini companies are small businesses and the owners are more than willing to help you through the process.

Connectors

Connectors are the sparkly bits that connect the parts of your suit together. You can have connectors on the straps at your neckline, between your cups and on the sides of your bottoms. Some companies also offer an option to have sparkly back connectors. I remember feeling really overwhelmed with all the options when I was selecting my suit, so I don't want you to feel that way! My advice for you is to look at what the pros are wearing and try to mimic that within your budget. Usually the straight, thick connectors are a safe bet. In the first edition of this book, I mentioned that the three tiered dangly connectors on the hip were popular. And while there are still top pros that wear them (India Paulino among others), the new suggestion is to avoid them because the dangly connectors cut off the length of the leg. It just goes to show you how subjective these things are and to really choose something that you love and feel confident in.

If you are on a tight budget this is one of the areas you can save money by choosing less expensive connectors. One other tip is to avoid choosing connectors that have small details. These have a tendency to break. Make sure you bring an emergency kit with safety pins on the day of the show for this reason.

Embellishments

Sequin vs. Bling? I say if you have the budget for it, go with bling, crystals pick up the light better than sequins. I also recommend choosing colored crystals that match the color of your suit. However, if you are only doing a local show and looking to save money sequins can look great too. One of my favorite suits that I own is a sequined one. Also, make sure you get good quality crystals as opposed to rhinestones. Crystals are finely cut pieces of glass or stone that catch light and really sparkle. If your suit maker says that they will embellish it with "rhinestones" that can mean anything including bits of dried glue. Trust me, the first suit I ever bought had rhinestones and it looked cheap and tacky. If you are going to spend the money on bling make sure they are quality crystals (Swarovski is one renowned brand of crystal).

Budget

Your competition bikini can be very expensive. If you are just getting started, no need to break the bank— you can find great suits for around $100 at some of the sites I have listed. You can also look around for used suits. Asking fellow competitors or your coach if they have gently used suits that you could buy or borrow will save you money. Suittrade.com and Divaexchange.com are two websites that facilitate the sale and purchase of used suits. Also if you have a budget in mind and see a suit that you really like outside of your budget, you can let the designer know about your budget and see if they can make something similar in your price range. Set yourself a budget and work from there, but remember good is not always cheap and cheap is not always good. You work hard on your physique, so make sure you are not cutting corners when it comes to presentation.

While it is possible to make your own suit, I don't recommend it unless you are a super talented seamstress. Chances are, the time you spend on making your suit is more valuable than the money you would have saved by purchasing a professionally created one.

Final Suit Advice

The competition bikini is a very important part of your competition package. Make sure you are presenting your best self. Even though I have given several guidelines, the choice is ultimately up to you so choose something that makes you feel amazing on your big day!

Competition Shoes

For the competition you will want a pair of clear high heel shoes. The heels should be between 4-6 inches high, with 5 inches being the average height. The shoe should NOT have a platform even if you are very short. There are a few styles to choose from but the two main brands are Ellie and Pleaser.

I have read that Ellie shoes are slightly wider than Pleaser shoes. I have slightly wider feet so I purchase Ellie's. Some of the reviews say to order up a half size, but I ordered a full size up (9) from my natural size (8) and they fit perfectly.

I also ordered the pair with the strap. Although the strap can visually break the line of your leg, it is clear so it really isn't that noticeable. It is more important that you are able to walk easily and confidently and I found the strap allowed me to do that. You can find a link to the exact shoe I purchased on my website at www.valeriewiest.com/shop.

Valerie Wiest

What are the judges looking for?

That is the million-dollar question. The difficult thing about physique competitions is that there are no exact measurements that the judges are looking for. It is a subjective sport and sometimes what the judges are looking for changes or varies depending on the judge. The NPC website states that the criteria for judging are as follows:

"Judges will be scoring competitors using the following criteria:

- *Balance and Shape*
- *Overall physical appearance including complexion, skin tone, poise and overall presentation."*

(NPC BIKINI DIVISION RULES, n.d.)

This does not make it very clear what the judges are looking for, however, if you spend time getting to know the industry there are some generally accepted guidelines as to what the expectations are.

Here are some key points that the judges are looking for in the bikini division:

- Balanced proportions (hourglass shape where body parts are evenly proportioned)
- Full, round glutes-This is a big one! Bikini is all about the booty! You are basically being judged from the waist down.
- Poise and personality.
- Feminine muscularity
- Who sucked the least- Rather than looking for who did the best, judges pick out flaws. It's easier to judge down based on flaws than to tally up everything a competitor did right.
- Hair, make up and suit should work together- make sure you choose something that feels like yourself, if you don't feel confident the judges will know.

28

- Use the competition tanner– Rookie mistake is showing up too light.
- Use good taste when it comes to your suit- Remember it is a family event.
- Leave hair down- there is no need to pull hair back in the back pose either.
- Smile- You'd be surprised how many girls don't do this on stage and what a big difference it makes in stage presence.

Posing

Posing is a huge component to your success as a competitor and each person should pose to suit their own body. In Bikini, there are only two poses: front and back. However, there are many different ways these can be executed. Not only are the poses themselves important, but your poise and charisma as you walk out on stage, transition and stand on the stage are big factors in your score as well.

I highly recommend going to a posing coach or at least having someone else critique your posing. Sometimes it's hard to see yourself objectively. Practice makes permanent and if you learn poses that don't suit your body that is what will stick in your mind. Taking pictures and videos of your posing can help too.

Make sure you practice your posing daily. When you get on stage there is a good chance that your mind will go blank so you want your posing routine to be so automatic that you don't even need to think about it.

On the day of your competition, pre-judging is where the actual judging takes place. The way it usually works is that each girl will be called to the stage to do her routine individually. The judges may give you a time frame for your posing routine, but don't freak out about it. It is better to spend too much time than too little time. A good rule of thumb is to hold each pose for 2 seconds (count in your head "one-Mississippi-two-Mississippi" so you don't rush). You will have a number badge so that the judges can identify you. Make sure this badge is visible or the judges will pass you by. Once you do your posing routine you will be escorted to the side of the stage while the next competitor goes. During this time, you will remain on the stage so it is important that you keep posing and smiling, as the judges are comparing you to the other competitors.

Once all of the competitors in your class have gone, it is time for call outs. The judge will call out the badge number of a few competitors. These competitors will come to the front of the stage for comparisons. This is where you really need to shine, because you are being directly compared to the other competitors. Sometimes the judges will just have you do a front and a back pose (they may do it multiple times). Other times they will have you walk to the back of the stage and then forward. If they do this, they are looking to see if anything jiggles. Walk SLOWLY on your tip toes so that nothing moves. They will also move competitors around which can indicate your placing.

In general, your placing in the competition is indicated by where you are placed on stage during call outs. The person in the center of the stage during first call outs will generally place first. The girls immediately to her left and right will place second and third and the girls to their left and right will be fifth and sixth and so on. Therefore, your goal is to be in the first group of girls they bring to the front of the stage and to be placed in the center of that group. This usually indicates that you will receive first place in the night show

In the night show, each girl gets to do a quick pose, depending on how many competitors there are, and awards are handed out. If you achieve first place in your class, your next goal will be to win the overall (first place for the whole bikini division). If you are looking to win the overall, you still have to bring your A-game to the night show, as the judges will be comparing you against the overall winners in the other height classes.

The bikini division is often the last group to go on stage, for this reason there will be a lot of time spent waiting around until you get to present yourself. Don't let this time stress you out. Bring music, an iPad or something else to help you relax and pass the time. This will help keep your spirits high, which will translate in the way you carry yourself on stage.

Here are some more guidelines for posing to help you take the show:

What NOT to do:

- DON'T move too much- The judges have to compare you to the other girls and if you are moving all over the place they can't judge you so they will move on to the next girl.
- DON'T look back in the back pose- When you look back you add movement and lose symmetry which makes it harder to judge.
- DON'T do the legs crossed back pose- Legs spread shows off glutes better.
- DON'T lose posture when you are on the side of the stage- Even when you are not front and center, you are being compared to the other girls on stage. Make sure you look your best at all times.
- DON'T Jiggle- If the judge makes you walk, it's to see if you jiggle. You DON'T want to jiggle, so make sure you walk smoothly. The best way to do this is to walk super slowly on your toes.
- DON'T copy figure poses

What to Do:

- Back pose- Toes point slightly out so that the line of your leg continues straight down to your toes, legs spread not too far but not too narrow, arch back as much as possible but don't bend forward (family show, not porn show remember?), hair should be down.
- Front pose- Legs spread, weight on one hip with torso twisted. Try twisting to different sides, staggering feet and twisting to different angles to find a pose that shows off your figure the best.

31

- Transitions and Walk- Should be smooth with good posture, confidence and sex appeal. Think: Victoria Secret Runway Model.
- Be authentic in your posing- Make a routine that works for you and that you feel comfortable with. Judges will know if you are being phony.
- Show off your assets- For example, if you have a long torso and short legs, pose to create the illusion of balance. It's up to you (and your coach if you have one) to find your strengths and weaknesses and pose in a way that highlights your strengths, while downplaying your weaknesses.
- Keep your eyes on the judges and make sure you smile to keep that connection with them.

Training

Now let's get to the fun stuff: training and nutrition! Wi.
competing I thought that training and nutrition would be ˌ
secret key to getting the perfect body. However, I quickly realizeˌ
wasn't a secret key. It's just hard work and applying some basic
principles. Your secret keys throughout this process will be discipline
and determination.

First, let's get one thing straight. Lifting weights is the most effective
way to sculpt your body. While you can't train to lose fat in certain spots,
you can train to build muscle in certain spots. Thus, by selectively
building muscle, while reducing all over body fat you can create the
athletic hourglass look that you are after.

The best way to build and maintain muscle is to lift heavy and train
often. For hypertrophy (building muscle), The American College of
Sports Medicine recommends a multiple set, high volume program
working at 6-12 repetition maximum with only 1-2 min. of rest between
sets. (Kraemer WJ, 2002)That means doing 2 or more sets and lifting a
weight heavy enough that you can do at least 6 repetitions, but no more
than 12. This strikes a balance between muscle tension and time under
tension, which is the key to building and maintaining muscle. While this
is a good guideline; training in different set and rep ranges can be
beneficial by affecting the development of different muscle fibers.
(Gerson E. Campos, 2002) Thus, for my sample training program, I stick
mostly to hypertrophy training, but add in some sets in different rep
ranges. Just know that the weight you are lifting should adjust with the
number of sets and reps you are doing so that by the last repetition in a
set you are just about at failure.

The bikini division is all about glutes, there will be a lot of the focus on
sculpting your glutes, and developing a nice glute-hamstring tie in. If you
look at the pro competitors you will notice that the hallmark of a pro is

upside down tear drop shaped glutes, with hamstrings that pop. ell defined quads and shoulder caps are also a requirement. Abs should be toned, but usually a "two-pack" is preferred to a completely ripped "six pack." Bikini is a softer look so extremely ripped or large muscles will be scored negatively.

That said, you really need at least some base of muscle mass to do well in a competition. It takes a lot longer to build muscle than it does to lose fat. If you are training for the first time, try focusing on building muscle at least one year before you decide to enter a competition. From there; however, it is your job to assess where you need to build muscle and where you need to lean down.

I do not believe in training for hours a day. That is one of the reasons I am writing this book. I think there are too many coaches out there that encourage their clients to do hours and hours of cardio and training setting them up for metabolic damage, overuse injuries, eating disorders and depression. You should be able to complete most of my workouts in about an hour with about 20-45min of additional cardio. You will also have one day off a week.

Days off are very important. Rest is when your body and muscles recover. Muscle recovery is when you also have muscle growth. If you are over training, you can end up sabotaging your results and slowing down your metabolism. That means sleeping enough and taking time off if you are sick too. I have been sick a couple times during training and my coach always encourages me to rest. If you try to push through your sickness you may end up prolonging the healing process.

In general, here is how I set up my training sessions: The first day of leg training is focused on glutes and calves, next I do an upper body day focused on biceps, triceps and shoulders. I take one day off of strength training in the middle of the week to just do plyometrics. Then, I have another leg day, this time focused on quads and hamstrings, another upper body day which is focused on chest and back and I close of the week off with one day focused on building up my weak spots: glutes, hamstrings and shoulders. I work in abs about one to two times a week and take one day completely off on the weekend. Since the look of bikini requires a small waist and since training your abs builds your abdominal muscles, you should avoid doing lots of ab work. You will build a strong core just by doing compound lifts like squats, deadlifts and lunges anyway.

I find that this upper/lower split allows me to hit muscle groups more often than the traditional 5-day split. This enables me to get more volume in each week, which will lead to more muscle growth in the long run. If you choose to structure your plan differently, make sure you give each muscle group time to recover before training it again.

The biggest mistake I see people make regarding training is just following a generic plan. Very few people have the glute development required for success in the bikini division without specifically training for it and some people build muscle easily in their quads and upper body while their glutes refuse to grow. Therefore, I think it is important that you train for your body type.

Training for Your Body Type

In order to decide on a training plan, you need to determine your physique's strengths and weaknesses. This is another place a coach can really be useful. A coach can objectively assess your body and help you improve your weaknesses with a custom plan. There are days when I look in the mirror and think my arms look like anacondas and there are other days when I look and I see two limp water hoses. My coach helps me to cut through my emotions and tells me objectively how I am progressing. A coach will also individualize your training program to meet your needs. You can find out more about my coach at www.JessicaJessie.com.

The majority of people will be starting out in one of two places: either over fat with an average amount of muscle mass or underweight, needing to build muscle while staying lean. Very rarely someone will have too much muscle, but I will address that too. Sometimes people will have too much muscle in one area and not enough in another. Since your goal is to balance out your physique each of these situations will require a different training plan.

The sample training program I provide in this book will work for most people who are already relatively proportioned and just need to lean down while maintaining or building a little muscle mass. However, with some small tweaks it can work for just about anyone.

Need to Lose Fat

Stick with the training program provided and decrease caloric intake or increase cardio if you see progress stall. When you lose weight, some of the weight is going to be muscle too, so you need to focus on losing fat while maintaining muscle in the right spots.

Need to Build Muscle

Stick with the training program provided and eat slightly more food and do slightly less cardio to avoid losing muscle.

Your goal is to maximize fat loss while minimizing muscle loss. A body recomposition is when your weight does not necessarily change, but your body fat percentage does. If you are already thin and just need to build muscle, this is the ideal situation. Eating a high protein diet with sufficient calories and lifting heavy weights will enable you to do this.

Need to Reduce Muscle

Decrease weight and number of sets and increase repetitions so that you maintain muscle tone without adding more mass. Add more cardio or decrease food if your progress stalls.

Overall Imbalanced

Lift heavy with more sets in the 6-12 rep range for the body parts you need to build muscle. Work in the higher repetition range with fewer sets and lower weight where you need to reduce size.

Valerie Wiest

Training Glutes Successfully

Because our modern lifestyle often has us sitting for hours each day with our glutes in the stretched position, many people have lost the ability to fire their glutes correctly. This makes training glutes more difficult, but it certainly won't stop you from building your backside. What tends to happen when glutes are underactive, is that the quads, or lower back take over when glutes are supposed to fire.

Here are a few tips to ensure that your glutes are firing during glute exercises. First, make sure you are using the mind-body connection. What I mean by that, is that you need to think about the exercise as you are doing it. When you are doing glute exercises ask yourself "where am I feeling this?" If you are not feeling glutes you will need to make an adjustment to your form.

To help activate your glutes more effectively here are some adjustments you can make to your form:

- Push through your heels- The backs of your legs are connected by fascia, nerves and connective tissue. By pushing through your heels you help to take the work out of your quads and put it more in your backside.
- Hip load instead of knee loading- When you are doing a squat or lunge make sure that your knees don't come past your toes. Send your hips back and think about putting the work in your glutes.
- Keep your core tight- When doing exercises like hip thrusts and kick backs that involve hip extension, make sure you are pulling your abs in with the same intensity that you are squeezing your glutes. This will ensure that the work goes into your glutes rather than into your lower back.

On the next page is an 8-week sample plan that you can use as the base for your training and tweak to meet your needs. You will want to lift heavy enough that by the last rep you are almost to failure. The final week of the show you can dial your weights back a little so that you are not sore on stage. You will have one rest day before your competition day.

Bikini Prep Workout Plan

Week 1-2

Lower Body: Glutes, Calves, Abs

4x15 Booty Pushdown on Assisted Pull-up Machine

4x10 Barbell Squat

4x 12 Smith Machine Lunge

4x12 Cable Kick Backs

4x12 Seated Calf Raise

4x15 Cable Crunches

Upper Body: Biceps, Triceps, Shoulders

4x12 Dumbbell Curls

4x12 Tricep Press Downs

4x12 Lateral Raise

4x10 Cable Curls

4x10 Arnold Press

4x10 Dumbbell Tricep Kick Back

4x8 Dumbbell Rear Delt Raise

4x8 Front Raise

Lower Body: Hamstrings, Quads

4x12 Leg Press

4x12 Machine Hamstring Curl

4x12 Leg Extensions

4x12 (each side) Step Ups

4x12 Deadlifts

Upper Body: Back, Chest

4x12 Wide Grip Lat Pull Down

4x12 Narrow Grip Row

4x12 Barbell Row

4x12 Barbell Chest press

4x12 Dumbbell Fly

Glutes and Shoulders (Weak Areas)

4x12 Barbell Glute Bridges

4x12 Barbell Hip Thrusts

4x12 Kettlebell Swings

4x12 Barbell Shoulder Press

4x12 Front Plate Raise

Plyometrics

Repeat 3 times 1 minute rest between sets

20x High Jumps

20x Narrow Jumps

20x Switch Jumps

20x Frog Jumps

Week 3-4

Lower Body: Glutes, Calves, Abs
4x20 Hip Thrusts

4x20 (each side) Single Leg Glute Bridge

4x20 Abductor machine

4x20 Adductor machine

4x20 (each side) Walking Weighted Lunges

4x20 Standing Calves

4x15 Stability Ball Knee tucks
Superset
4x15 Stability Ball Crunches

Upper Body: Biceps, Triceps, Shoulders
4x12 Hammer Curls

4x12 Dumbbell Overhead Triceps Press

4x12 Dumbbell Shoulder Press

4x10 Concentration Curl

4x10 Skull Crushers

4x10 Rear Delt Cable Extension

4x8 Plate Shoulder Raise

Lower Body: Hamstrings, Quads
4x20 Stability Ball Hamstring Curls

4x20 Narrow Stance Hack Squat

Secrets of the Bikini Competitor

Valerie Wiest

4x20 (each side) TRX Lunge (or Bulgarian Split Squat if No TRX)

4x20 (each side) Kettlebell Single Leg Deadlifts

4x20 Leg Extension

Upper Body: Back, Chest, Shoulders

4x10 (each side) Single Arm Lat Pull Down

4x10 T-Bar Row

4x10 Dumbbell row

4x10 Dumbbell chest press

4x10 Pec Deck

4x10 Push-ups

Glutes and Shoulders (Weak Areas)

4x10 Barbell Squats

4x10 (each side) Barbell Lunge (Step your leg out as far as possible)

4x10 Barbell Shoulder Press

4x10 Weighted Donkey Kicks

4x15 Cable Front Raise

4x10 Rear Delt Fly on Pec Deck

Plyometrics

Repeat 3 times 1 minute rest between sets

20 Split squats

20 Pop Squats

20 Weighted Wide Jumps

Secrets of the Bikini Competitor

20 Weighted Narrow Jumps

20 Mountain Climbers

Week 5-6

Lower Body: Glutes, Calves, Abs
6x6 (each side) Single Leg Reverse Hack Squat

8x8 (each side) Butt Blaster Machine

6x 6 Barbell Squats

4x10 Barbell Calf Raises

6x6 Reverse Smith Machine Leg Press

4x20 Bicycle Crunch

Upper Body: Biceps, Triceps, Shoulders
6x6 Single Arm Cable Curl

4x10 Incline Dumbbell Curl

6x6 Overhead Tricep Cable Press

6x6 Dumbbell Skull Crushers

5x8 Arnold Press

5x8 High Cable Rope Pull

6x6 Cable Lateral Raise

Lower Body: Hamstrings, Quads
6x6 (each side) Single Leg Lying Hamstring Curl

6x6 (each side) Single Leg Extension

6x6 (each side) Single Leg Press

4x15 Glute-Ham Raise

6x6 Hex bar Deadlifts

Upper Body: Back, Chest, Shoulders
6x6 Cable Row

6x6 Single Arm Dumbbell Row

5x5 Assisted Pull-up

5x5 Assisted Dips

4x12 Cable Fly

4x12 Push-ups

Glutes and Shoulders (Weak Areas)
4x10 (each side) Weighted Bulgarian Split Squat

4x10 (each side) Barbell Side Lunge

4x10 (each side) Cable Kick Backs

4x10 Reverse Hyperextensions

4x10 Dumbbell Lateral Raise

4x10 Dumbbell Rear Delt Raise

Plyometrics
Repeat 4 times 1 minute rest between sets

20x Bench Hops (Both feet jump on then off in a straddle)

20x Weighted Split Lunge

20x Weighted Pop Squats

Valerie Wiest

20x Wide Jump Hold 5 sec

Week 7-8

Lower Body: Glutes, Calves, Abs

4x12 (each side) Smith Machine Lunge

4x12 (each side) Side Leg Press Machine

4x12 (each side) Cable Kick Backs & Abduction

3x10 Kettle Bell Swings

3x10 Leg Press with Toes Hanging Off the Top (targets glutes)

3x10 Leg Press Calf Raises

3x10 Decline Crunches

Upper Body: Biceps, Triceps, Shoulders

3x21 21's

3x10 Alternating Bicep Curl

3x10 Plate overhead Triceps Extension

3x10 Cable Straight Bar Triceps Pushdown

3x10 Machine Lateral Raise

3x10 Barbell Front Raises

3x10 Dumbbell Incline Rear Delt Y-raises

Lower Body: Hamstrings, Quads

3x10 Stiff Leg Dead lifts
Superset
3x20 Regular Jumps

Secrets of the Bikini Competitor

Valerie Wiest

3x10 Weighted TRX Lunge (or Bulgarian Split Squat if No TRX)
Superset
3x20 Frog Jumps

3x10 TRX Pistol Squat (or regular pistol squat if no TRX)
Superset
3x20 Split Squat

3x10 Leg Press
Superset
3x20 Narrow Jump

Upper Body: Back, Chest, Shoulders
3x10 Close Grip Lat Pull Down

3x10 Wide Grip Cable Rows

3x15 Push-ups

3x15 Pull Overs

3x10 Dumbbell Flys

3xAMRAP Pull-ups

Glutes and Shoulders (Weak Areas)
4x10 Barbell Squat

4x10 Barbell Sumo Squat

4x10 (each side) TRX Reverse Lunge or Bulgarian Split Squat

4x10 Hyperextensions

4x10 Arnold Press

4x10 Cable Rear Delt Raises

Secrets of the Bikini Competitor

Valerie Wiest

Plyometrics

Repeat 5 times 1 minute rest between sets

20x Grasshoppers

20x Frog Jumps

20x Wide Plie Jumps

20x Narrow Jumps

Week of Show

Lower Body: Glutes, Calves, Abs

3x15 Glute Bridge with 45lb Plate

3x15 Barbell Squats

3x15 Abductor

3x15 Adductor

3x15 Hip Thrusts

3x15 Standing Calf Raise

3x20 Deadbugs

Upper Body: Biceps, Triceps, Shoulders

3x10 Barbell Curl

3x10 Barbell Skull Crusher

3x10 Barbell Front Raise

3x10 Dumbbell Lateral Raise

3x10 Dumbbell Bicep Curl

3x10 Dumbbell Rear Delt Raise

3x15 Bench Dips

Lower Body: Hamstrings, Quads

3x10 Single Leg Hamstring Curl
Super Set
3x10 Single Leg, Leg Extension

3x10 Single Leg Kettle Bell Deadlift
Superset
3x10 Single Leg, Leg Press

3x10 Narrow Hack Squat
Superset
3x10 Reverse Hack Squat Straight Leg Deadlift

Upper Body: Back, Chest, Shoulders

3x10 (each side) Single Arm Lat Pull Down

3x10 (each side) Single Arm Cable Row

3x10 (each side) Single Arm Dumbbell Row

3x10 (each side) Single Arm Dumbbell Press

3x10 Cable Cross Overs

Cardio

The cardio you do for your bikini competition prep needs to build up your booty, not flatten it. Low resistance cardio on the elliptical and running on the treadmill with no incline will give you a flat butt. Below are some sample programs that I like to use when I am training for a bikini competition. I kept the duration between 20-30 min. I recommend doing cardio 4 times a week. If you are strict with your diet this should be enough. If you find yourself hitting a plateau, increasing your cardio slightly can help. I don't recommend going over 1 hour of cardio

High Intensity interval training is most effective at burning fat, so these programs are designed to give you bursts of intensity. (Angelo Tremblay, 1994)

Stair Master
Repeat 2-3 times

4 min Level 8 w/kickback

1 minute Level 15

4 min Level 12

1 minute Level 15

Treadmill
Repeat 2-3 times

Incline 5-10

2 min walking lunges 2mph

2 min walking backwards 3mph

1 min run at 6mph

1 min side skip left 2mph

2 min walking lunges with kick backs 1.5mph

1 min side skip right 2mph

1 min run at 6mph

Sprints

10x Sprint 50 yards 30 sec rest

Diet

Diet is an essential part of your training. What you eat will make or break your physique. I often hear that training is 80% diet and 20% exercise and I really believe this to be true. To get the physique you want, you are going to have to follow a very strict diet plan. In the beginning, it may feel like you are eating a lot of food but as your metabolism adjusts, you may feel intense hunger. It's going to be up to you to push through that feeling of hunger and stay dedicated to your training.

Nutrition can be a tricky subject. There are so many different philosophies out there and what works for one person may not work as well for another. I believe in eating healthy, unprocessed foods as much as possible. I am also against starvation diets which is the basis of many "competition coaches'" plans. If you have a coach who is telling you to eat less than 1200 calories a day, drop them immediately.

Most bodies need at least 1200 calories to function and with the intense type of training you will be doing you need to fuel your body even while you are trying to lean down. I used to believe that less is more when it came to calories but now I know that when your body is not getting enough fuel to survive, it will feed off of your muscle, destroying all of your hard work at the gym.

Many bikini competition programs offer a cookie cutter diet and while people may see results, the program may not be the most effective for their body. Following the wrong meal plan can lead to things like metabolic damage, depression and eating disorders. Therefore, in my diet program, I teach you how to create your own meal plan that is customized for your body.

To find a meal plan that is right for your body, the first thing you will want to do is calculate your caloric needs. You can do this on my website at **www.valeriewiest.com/calorie-calculator** or you can follow the

Harris Benedict formula by entering your information into the following equation:

Women BMR = 447.593 + (9.247 x weight in kg) + (3.098 x height in cm) - (4.330 x age in years)

Then multiply the result you got by your activity factor:

Little to no exercise   Daily kilocalories needed = BMR x 1.2
Light exercise (1–3 days per week)   Daily kilocalories needed = BMR x 1.375
Moderate exercise (3–5 days per week)   Daily kilocalories needed = BMR x 1.55
Heavy exercise (6–7 days per week)   Daily kilocalories needed = BMR x 1.725
Very heavy exercise (twice per day, extra heavy workouts) = BMR x 1.9

As a side note, there are also wearable devices that keep track of calories burned each day (Fitbit, Jawbone, etc.). I have found these tools to be helpful in calculating my energy expenditure, but not always entirely accurate. For me, these devices tended to overestimate my caloric burn slightly. For example, the device would say I had burned 2700 calories in a day when I was maintaining my weight on 2300 calories. Still, the comparison aspect was helpful: I could tell which days and what activities caused me to burn more calories overall.

Once you have calculated your caloric needs, you need to decide how many calories to cut to reach your goal within the allotted amount of time. You can go back to your body fat percentage goal (8-12% is ideal for competition). If your goal is to lose 1% body fat per week and you weigh 140 lbs., then you want to lose 1.4 lbs of body fat per week. Since 1lb of body fat is approximately 3500 calories, you will need to cut 4900 calories from your diet per week. That is approximately a 700 calorie reduction per day. The equation would look like this:

((Weight in Pounds x Percent Body Fat to Lose x 3500)/ # of Weeks to Goal /7 = Calories to Reduce Intake per Day

Just wanted to remind you that you can check out my website for a free calculator at http://www.valeriewiest.com/calorie-calculator to do it the easy way if your head is still spinning from all this math.

To me, reducing calories by 700 a day seems a bit severe. I prefer to set a smaller goal in body fat reduction, only reducing calories by 200-500 per day and then lowering my calories further if needed when progress stalls. This type of prep takes longer but it is more comfortable and will allow you to keep your metabolism from slowing down drastically in response to the sudden reduction of food intake. I also find that people who diet severely often end up rebounding worse once the competition is over. We'll talk more about that in the Post Competition section.

Once you have your calorie requirements you should calculate how those calories will be broken down into macros. "Macros" is short for macronutrients which have three different categories: protein, carbohydrates (carbs) and fat.

Acceptable Macronutrient Distribution Ranges for Adults (as a percentage of Calories) are as follows:
Protein: 10-35%
Fat: 20-35%
Carbohydrate: 45-65%
Fiber recommendation for females age 19-50 is 25g per day

(Institute of Medicine of the National Academies, 2005)

I have created a free calculator at my website www.valeriewiest.com/macro-calculator/ to help you calculate these values.

I find that a higher protein and relatively low fat and carb diet is the most effective way to lose fat. Research supports this position. (Carol S. Johnston, 2004) Protein has a higher thermic effect of food which means that it takes the body more calories to process protein than to process fat or carbs. Additionally, eating more protein leads to higher satiety, which means you will be feeling less hungry through your diet. (Crovetti R, 1998) Finally, since protein provides the building blocks for muscle, by consuming higher levels of protein, your body is primed to conserve and even build muscle while burning fat. (Heather J. Leidy, 2007)

For this reason, I recommend structuring meals around the ratio 35% protein, 20% fat and 45% carbs. This maximizes the protein ratio within the recommended daily levels. To convert these ratios in to calories, simply calculate the percentage of your daily calories for each macronutrient. To calculate the number of grams of each macronutrient that you should be eating based on your caloric requirements, divide the number of calories per macronutrient by 4 for carbohydrates and protein (there are approximately 4 calories for each gram of carb or protein) and 9 for fats (there are approximately 9 calories per each gram of fat). Please remember that these equations including the caloric needs you calculated are approximate and your plan should be adjusted based on your results and how you feel. If this is confusing, don't forget that you can use the free calculator on my website www.valeriewiest.com/macro-calculator/ to help your calculate these values.

Step-By-Step DIY Diet

Since I know that last section can be a bit intense I wanted to include a quick step by step guide to creating your own meal plan guidelines:

1. Calculate your caloric needs by plugging your information into the "Daily Calorie Requirements Calculator" on my website: www.valeriewiest.com/calorie-calculator
2. Scroll down on the same page of my website and use the results you just got to calculate how many calories you need to eat to reach your goal weight or body fat loss using either the "Calorie Requirements for Fat Loss Calculator" or the "Calorie Requirements for Weight Loss Calculator."
3. Calculate your goal macronutrient breakdown by going to my website: http://valeriewiest.com/macro-calculator/ and plugging in your calorie requirements for fat or weight loss.

Pre and Post Workout Nutrition

In Drs. John Ivy and Robert Portman's 2004 book *Nutrient Timing*, they discuss how to optimize the intake of certain nutrients at specific times during a 24 hour cycle to maximize muscle growth while minimizing muscle damage. The 24 hour cycle is broken down into 3 phases:

1. Energy Phase- This is your workout. During this phase, or slightly before, you want to eat a high carbohydrate, high antioxidant meal with a small amount of protein. Doing this, helps to spare glycogen, spare muscle tissue, maintain immune function, and minimize the damage of cortisol.
2. Anabolic Phase- This is 45 minutes post workout. A 3:1 or 4:1 carbohydrate to protein ratio is recommended. This stimulates insulin, which increases blood flow thereby helping to speed the elimination of metabolic waste. It also blunts cortisol release, replenishes glycogen stores, and helps to stimulate muscle synthesis.
3. Growth Phase-This is the remaining 18-24 hours in your day. This phase has two segments: The rapid growth segment (1-5

hours post workout) and the sustained segment (5 hours post workout until next workout). During the rapid growth segment small feedings of carbohydrate and protein every 1-2 hours can help maintain the anabolic (muscle building) phase and further support muscle synthesis and glycogen replenishment. During the sustained segment it is important to eat enough protein to maintain a positive nitrogen balance to support and stimulate protein synthesis. Eating an adequate amount of carbohydrates and fats is also important to avoid using amino acids (the building blocks of protein) as fuel.

(John & Portman, 2004)

To sum this up, pre and post workout nutrition will focus on higher carbohydrates with small amounts of protein to encourage protein and muscle synthesis and to replenish glycogen stores. The rest of the day will be focused on getting adequate protein, fat and carbohydrates.

What to Eat

Now that you have calculated macronutrients you are ready to set up your meal plan but first let's talk about what food you should be eating. IIFYM is a popular dieting strategy lately, which stands for "if it fits your macros." The idea is that if you can hit the macros (macronutrients) you just calculated, you can eat whatever you want. The reason I don't like this approach is because it doesn't account for fiber or micronutrients-- vitamins and minerals that are essential for healthy functioning. You also may end up feeling super hungry if you are not eating healthy, unprocessed food. This is because the caloric density of food is often higher with processed food, which means that you get less food for more calories. The result—you will be HANGRY. Personally, I have experienced better results from eating whole unprocessed foods rather than eating the same number of macronutrients from protein bars and other processed sources.

That said, I think that IIFYM gets it right in the fact that you can incorporate a treat in to your diet every once in a while if it fits into your macros. I also think you can branch out of the traditional "bro foods" of sweet potatoes, chicken, tilapia, broccoli and asparagus to other healthy foods. For example, fruits are a taboo topic for some competitors, but I think eating fruit is totally fine. Although fruit contains sugar it, also contains fiber and water, which helps slow down digestion and stabilize blood sugar. Fruit can also be a great choice pre-workout when you want something high in carbohydrates and antioxidants.

During competition prep you are going to be doing an intense amount of training with a reduced amount of food. Because of this, you want to make sure that you are eating nutrient dense foods. Nutrient dense foods are usually foods that are as unprocessed as possible. This way, you can make sure you are getting quality fuel for your body. Here is a list of some healthy foods that I eat during competition (and during regular life too):

Protein:
Chicken breast
Lean ground chicken
Turkey breast
Lean ground turkey
Lean steak
Tilapia
Salmon
Swordfish
Sea bass
Mahi-mahi
Grilled calamari
Shrimp
Scallops

Cottage cheese

Greek yogurt

Whey isolate Protein powder

Egg whites

Whole eggs

Carbohydrates:

Leafy greens

Green beans

Asparagus

Brussels sprouts

Brown rice

Potatoes

Sweet potatoes

Squash

Bell peppers

Onions

Mushrooms

Oatmeal

Quinoa

Water melon

Berries

Mango

Pineapple

Banana

Apple

Ezekiel bread

Fats:

Fish oil

Flax oil

Walnuts

Almonds

Pistachios

Cashews

Almond milk

Vinaigrette

Olive oil

Coconut oil

Avocado

Almond butter

Of course, this is just a sample of some of the foods that I eat, but you get the idea, right? On the next page are 3 sample daily meal plans. The meal plan is based on a diet of approximately 1600 calories with 35% protein 20% fat and 45% carbs. Feel free to make your own meal plans using these guidelines or adjust the calories/macros to meet your goals.

My meal plans have six meals each day. Eating regularly helps to keep your blood sugar stable and helps regulate hunger. It also helps you to maintain energy while keeping your metabolism stoked. (Hamid R Farshchi, 2005) However, if having six meals a day just doesn't work for your lifestyle, it's ok to do slightly more or slightly fewer. Meal frequency does not have that big of an affect as long as you are meeting your macronutrient goals.

If you start to reach a plateau, it is usually because of your diet. If you notice that you are not progressing as quickly as you would like, adjust your calories and macros accordingly. Conversely, if you have no energy and are dropping weight too quickly you may need to increase your calories.

Don't forget to download my free meal prep guide at www.bikinimealprep.com for tips on how to make preparing your food and planning your meals easier.

Sample Meal Plans

Diet Plan 1:

Meal 1

2 Whole Eggs

1/3 Cup Oatmeal

1 T Flax oil

Meal 2

1 slice of Ezekiel or P28 Bread

1T Almond butter

Meal 3

6 oz. Chicken Breast

0.25 oz. Walnuts

1 cup Leafy Greens

4 oz. Sweet Potato

Meal 4

6oz Salmon

12 Spears Asparagus

Meal 5 (Pre-workout)

Fruit Smoothie:

1 cup Unsweetened Almond Milk

0.5 cup Frozen Pineapple

0.5 cup Frozen Mango

1 Scoop Protein Powder

Meal 6 (Post workout)

1 Scoop Protein Powder, 1 Banana or Small Apple

1651 Calories

139 Carbs, 51 Fat, 162 Protein

Diet Plan 2:

Meal 1

Omelet:

3 Egg whites

1 Whole Egg

¼ cup Veggies of Choice (i.e. tomatoes, broccoli, onions, bell peppers)

1/3 cup Oatmeal

1 T Flax Oil

Meal 2

2 cups Spaghetti squash

1T Coconut Oil

Meal 3

6 oz. Chicken

12 Spears Asparagus

0.5 T Coconut Oil

4 oz. Sweet Potato

Meal 4

6 oz. Lean Ground Turkey

1 Cup Broccoli

Meal 5 (Pre-workout)

6 oz. Chicken Breast

1 cup Leafy Greens

1 Banana

Meal 6 (Post workout)

1 Scoop Protein Powder, 1 cup of Blueberries or Strawberries

1673 Calories

129 Carbs, 48 Fat, 160 Protein

Diet Plan 3:

Meal 1

4 Egg Whites

Valerie Wiest

1/3 Cup Oatmeal

1 T Flax Oil

Meal 2

6 oz. Chicken Breast

4 oz. Sweet potato

1 Cup Leafy Greens

1T Almond butter

Meal 3

6 oz. Chicken Breast

1 T Low Calorie Dressing (45 calories or less)

1 cup Leafy Greens

4 oz. Sweet Potato

Meal 4

6 oz. Chicken Breast

12 Spears Asparagus

4 oz. Sweet Potato

Meal 5 (Pre-workout)

1 Medium Banana

1 Scoop Protein Powder

Meal 6 (Post workout)

1 Cup Fat Free Chocolate Milk

Secrets of the Bikini Competitor

Valerie Wiest

1636 calories

157 Carbs, 37 Fat, 166 Protein

Supplements

In general, I feel like people take way more supplements than are necessary. However, there are a few supplements that I recommend while training for a competition.

- **Multivitamin**- This is basically to close the nutritional gaps that may be caused by eating at a caloric deficit. Check with your doctor to make sure that you are not overdosing on any vitamins in your supplement regimen.

- **Vitamin C**- Vitamin C is an antioxidant and helps with immune support. You will be training intensely at a caloric deficit making your body susceptible to illness. I also find that taking 1000-2000mg/day of vitamin C helps me to ward off colds and other sicknesses, and/or lessens their severity.

- **Calcium/Magnesium**- Calcium and magnesium work together. Calcium is essential for maintaining the strength and health of bones and teeth and magnesium is responsible for the production of certain enzymes. A lack of magnesium can lead to muscle cramps and poor sleep. To get my daily dose of calcium and magnesium, I like drinking CALM (a powder supplement) before bed.

- **Flax Oil**- It's important that you get healthy fats in your diet. Healthy fats help regulate hormones and also help improve the quality of skin, nails and joints. I love the flavored kind by Barlean's in my oatmeal.

- **Glucosamine**- This is a supplement for joint health. While the research has not been conclusive on the benefits of this supplements for healthy humans, I find that Glucosamine helps my joints (particularly my knees) feel better during intense training.

- **Glutamine**- Glutamine is an amino acid that helps with muscle recovery. Some glutamine will be in your whey protein, so this is an optional supplement.

- **Whey Protein**- Protein helps boost your metabolism because of its high thermic effect of food (how many calories you spend on digestion). Whey protein in particular, is well absorbed by the body and has been proven to increase muscle synthesis when taken before and after workouts. (Cribb, 2006) . For my competitions I used Dymatize ISO-100 because it is a whey isolate low in sugar and calories.

- **Creatine**- Creatine is a naturally occurring substance in your body that is used for energy production. When you supplement with creatine you can increase muscle cell volume, promote lean mass, and reduce recovery time. (JS Volek, 1999) However, some people find that creatine can have a bloating effect, so if you find this to be true, you may not want to use it. I don't have issues with bloating and my favorite brand is Con-Cret. The pineapple flavor is the best!

- **Fat Burner**- Many coaches recommend a fat burner as a requirement. I, however, don't believe that to be the case. Most fat burners work by using stimulants to increase your metabolic rate. The effect this actually has on how many calories you burn is debatable. Fat burners can also make some people feel jittery or sick to their stomach. During my competitions I did not use a fat burner.

There are many supplements out there, but I think keeping the supplements minimal is the best approach. The dose you take for each supplement will depend on your goals, body composition and size. Talk to your doctor before you add any supplements into you training program. You can find links to the supplements I mentioned on my website at www.valeriewiest.com/shop.

Valerie Wiest

Hair and Make-up

Hair and make-up are an important part of your look on the big day. Part of what you will be judged on is your "overall physical appearance including complexion, skin tone, poise and overall presentation" so how you present yourself really matters. (NPC BIKINI DIVISION RULES, n.d.) In this section I will discuss the ins and outs of competition hair and make-up, but be sure to check out my interview with professional competition hair and make-up artist Christy Tate towards the end of the book.

While you can definitely pay someone to do your hair and make-up, these services can run around $300. If you are interested in saving money, it may be worth learning how to do it yourself. However, if the idea of doing your own hair and make-up on show day stresses you out, definitely hire a professional. If you are going to pay someone to do it, make sure it is someone who has done competition make-up and hair before. Competition make-up and hair are definitely different from everyday make-up and you don't want to stand out in a bad way. If you choose to use the show sponsored make-up or hair artist, make sure their style matches yours, and that they customize each look so that their clients don't end up looking like clones of each other. The goal is to bring out YOUR best features to help YOU stand out.

Hair

If you are interested in doing your own hair here are my tips.

In general judges prefer two main looks for hair: straight hair, or beachy voluminous waves ala Victoria's Secret models. Either way, your hair should look healthy and youthful, not fried and dried. If you are in doubt, go with straight hair. In my opinion, it is safer and easier to do.

I have also seen girls with short edgy hairstyles do well, so if that is your style, go with it. However, note that there are very few pros with short hair and I am sure that is not a coincidence!

One of the other things you will want to consider is extensions. You can use extensions if you have short hair, or if you just want to add more volume to your long hair. Remember, you will be on stage so everything needs to be a little more dramatic in order to catch the judges' attention. Most competitors use extensions.

I got my extensions from my hair stylist. I bought the kind that clip into your hair which makes it super easy to install them. My stylist also cut and dyed the extensions for me. If you don't have a stylist you can go to, try looking at beauty supply stores or online. You don't have to have top of the line extensions but they should blend in with your hair and look as natural as possible. Professional competition hair stylist, Cristy Tate, recommends Remy human hair extensions.

As I mentioned, the two hair styles I recommend for competing are:

- Straight Shiny Hair
- Voluminous (Victoria Secret Style) Waves

For straight hair, it is relatively straight forward. The night before your competition you will want to blow dry your hair using a heat protectant. On the day of your competition, put a volumizing heat protecting mousse on your hair.

Separate your hair into manageable chunks, clipping it out of the way. Select a section from the bottom of your head near the nape of your neck. To maintain some volume, place the straightener about a half inch from your roots and slide the straightener down your hair moving at a smooth even pace. Repeat with the sections on the bottom and middle half of your head, leaving just the hair at your crown.

For the remaining sections at the top of your head, place the iron as close to your scalp as you can and slide the iron straight out from your head. Finish with a shine spray.

For your Victoria Secret soft curls, use hot rollers. I used a kit from Babybliss, you can find it on my website at www.valeriewiest.com/shop, but you can use any set of large hot rollers. Avoid small rollers, because it will make the curls look too tight and prom-like. Once your rollers are hot you are going to separate a 2" section right down the center of your head (sort of like a Mohawk). You will use about 3-4 large rollers for this section, curling the hair away from your face. Next you will do the sides, you will use about 3-4 large or medium rollers on each side, curling your hair away from your face. For each section you curl, comb the hair straight, then, tease the roots, and spray with a firm hold hair spray. I like Big Sexy Hair firm hold spray for this. Once your entire head is in rollers, spray the hair spray all over and wait until your rollers cool. After the rollers have cooled, take them out, flip your head upside down and give your hair another spritz of hair spray. Flip your head back up and tousle your hair until you have soft voluminous waves.

If you are curling your hair you will want to leave the rollers in as long as possible so that your hair does not go flat.

You will also want to make sure that you have a hair clip so that you can keep your hair off your back, which will be covered in fake tan and oil.

Make-up

Now let's talk make-up! It's fun to get glammed up but if you are not used to doing your own make-up, it can be intimidating. If you feel totally intimidated, hire a professional. However, if you are comfortable doing your own make-up, learning how to do your competition look can save you money. Remember, because you will be on stage and the bright lights will wash you out, everything will need to be more dramatic.

Here is a list of the make-up items and colors I used for my competition. You will need the same items, but choose colors that match your personality and complexion. I am listing all MAC make-up items because this is what I use. I am sure that some items could be substituted for cheaper, non-brand items:

Foundation: Pro Longwear NC45 (Take note, this shade will work for most people to get dark enough to match your tan)

Foundation Primer (you need this for your foundation to last all day)

Brow Pencil: Strawberry Blonde

Brow Gel: Clear

Blush: Breath of Plum

Lip Primer (optional)

Lip Liner: Half Red

Lip Stick: Sheen Supreme

Lip Gloss: Date Night

Eyeliner Stick and Pot: BlackTrack

Eye Base: Painterly

Eye Shadow 4 shades:

1 Bright for lash line: Crème De Violet

1 Dark for outer crease: Haux

1 Even Darker for deepening outer crease: Shadowy Lady

1 Light for high lighter: Naked Lunch

False Lashes #36

Lash Glue

You will also need brushes. I found a good deal on brushes on Amazon. You can find a link to the set I bought on my website www.valeriewiest.com/shop. While the large brushes in the set I bought shed, the smaller brushes worked great, and that's really all you will need the set for.

A couple of tips for your make-up:

1. Stage make-up is way different than regular make-up. You need it to be dramatic to be visible under the bright stage lights.
2. Don't go too matchy-matchy. Your eye shadow shouldn't match your suit unless it is black.
3. Silver and black tones look classier than bright colors when it comes to eye shadow.
4. Fake lashes are a must! Even if you think you have great lashes, the stage lights will wash them out. However, be careful about using fake lashes that are too full, as they can create odd shadows on your face.
5. Make sure you match your foundation to your tan. It should be no more than a shade or two lighter than your tan. Having a white face and a tan body is a big rookie mistake
6. If you are getting a spray tan, don't let them tan your face. Your foundation will make your face match the rest of your body. If you spray your face, your make-up tends to look muddy.

Here are the steps I followed for my make-up look:

1. Clean and lotion your skin, apply the primer all over your face.

2. Highlight the contours of your face with foundation or concealer around eyebrows to give them shape, in the creases between your nose and cheeks, at your cupid's bow, and around the corners of your mouth.

3. Use your brow pencil to lightly fill in your brows.

4. Brush your brow gel on your eyebrows to keep them in place.

5. Brush your eye base on your lid.

6. Use your pot liner and a liner brush to work your liner into the tear line of your top and bottom lid. Outline your entire lid with the liner and use your pencil liner to help define this line.

7. Dab your bright color eye shadow along your lash line.

8. Make a sideways "V" shape from the crease of your eye to the corners of your eyes using your dark shadow.

9. Re-enforce this shape with your darkest shadow.

10. Use your highlighter eye shadow just below the arch of your brow and dab a little at the inside corner of your eye

11. Use a make-up wipe to wipe off any extra shadow below or around your eyes.

12. Use your lash glue to lightly line the top edge of your false lashes. Place the lashes on your lid, as close to your lash line as possible.

13. Lightly line your lip with your lip liner (it should match your lipstick) I find that it helps to dot around your lip line lightly and then connect the dots.

14. Fill your lips in with lipstick.

15. Apply your Foundation with a kabuki style brush, dabbing it on for an air brush effect. Blend foundation into neck and ears.

16. Brush blush on the apples of your cheeks.

17. Apply lip gloss.

Jewelry

The rules state that competitors can wear jewelry. For the most part this means one or two bracelets, earrings and a ring or two. Do NOT wear a necklace, as It tends to break up the line of your body.

Jewelry should be large and bling-y but not too crazy. You want to catch the attention of the judges without distracting from your physique. You can find inexpensive crystal jewelry at costume jewelry stands in the mall or online. Of course, you can also buy Swarovski jewelry if you have an unlimited budget.

You can find a link to examples of pieces of jewelry that will work for your competition on my website www.valeriewiest.com/shop.

Ultimately the jewelry is not that important at the local level, so don't stress out too much about finding the "perfect" piece.

Tanning

Let's talk tan! If you ever wondered why bikini athletes have to get such dark tans, it's because the bright stage lights wash you out and a rich tan helps emphasize the curves of your muscles. Not being tan enough is a rookie mistake, so I highly recommend using the tanning services sponsored by the competition to ensure that you get a dark, even color. Protan, Liquid Sun Rayz and Jan Tana are a few well known and quality providers of spray tans.

For many athletes, tanning starts well before the day of the show in tanning beds. While many competitors feel this is the only way to go, I am against tanning beds. My aunt had skin cancer and I have also seen firsthand how tanning prematurely ages your skin. Next time you go to the tanning salon, check out the forehead wrinkles on the 20-something well-tanned girl at the reception desk. No thanks!

However, that's totally a personal choice (although for your health and well-being I hope I have convinced you otherwise). Most tanning companies also warn against tanning beds, because the resulting peeling, dry skin will ruin your spray tan. If you do decide to bake yourself, build up a base tan and then go once a week to maintain.

If I've brought you over to the pale side with me, you are going to need to get really dark with the spray tan and do a good job of camouflaging your face with make-up. You will need at least two to three coats of dark tan. This is another reason I recommend using the sponsored spray tan company. First of all, it is very convenient. Secondly, they really know what they are doing and can help ensure that you get a dark even tan. They also provide little extras like bikini bite (which glues your suit in place so that it won't ride up in your hoo-ha) and glaze (to make your body slightly shiny so that your muscles pop).

Secrets of the Bikini Competitor

Valerie Wiest

Usually the tanning companies offer two packages: one with a set number of tans and one with unlimited tans. If you are pale like me, make sure you get a package of at least 3 tans. If you are already dark, you can probably get away with 2 coats, but may want to go for 3 coats just to make sure you are dark enough. More than 3 coats is probably over kill so don't waste your money.

The tan is probably my least favorite part about competing. It is sticky, smelly and gets on everything. Not to mention that you can't shower and have to be really careful to avoid messing it up.

Here are a couple of tips to keep your tan looking fresh. First of all, you will want to wear very loose clothing and definitely NO spandex or workout gear once your tan has been applied. You will also want to avoid wearing underwear and a bra once you have been sprayed. Make sure you have these loose clothes with you when you go to your tanning appointment.

The next tip would be to keep well covered. One night I wore a Henley top with the buttons open at the front and I woke up with a big hand print on my chest where I had let my hand rest.

Also, be aware that the tan can and probably will stain any white cloth or clothing that it comes in contact with. If you are staying at a hotel make sure your check with the hotel about their policy regarding stains on sheets as some hotels will make you pay for damaged bed clothes. If they charge for stains, bring your own bedding.

You will also need to be really careful about getting water on yourself so that the tan doesn't run. This is particularly important when you go to the bathroom. Sorry to get graphic, but I find that hovering above the seat and going slowly is the best way to prevent pee streaks. I have seen and tried other methods such as the "go girl" (a portable urinal type device for women), the hole in the bottom of a cup, and the toilet paper on the seat, but I have found them all to be slightly more accident prone.

Another important aspect of the spray tan is preparing the skin so that the tan will appear even. In the Competition Countdown section I tell you exactly what to do to get the perfect tan.

If you decide to go the DIY route and apply your tan at home, I highly recommend using one of the tanning products provided by one of the major companies that offer competition tanning. This is because tanners made for the general population will not get you dark enough for your show. The brands I recommend are Protan, Liquid Sun Rayz and Jan Tana. Follow their directions for their product.

Valerie Wiest

Competition Countdown

12-8 weeks before: Hire Coach and start diet and exercise plan.
6 weeks before: Register for the show and order suit.
4 weeks before: Schedule spray tan.
2 weeks before: Get hair colored and cut if necessary.
Start applying lotion all over your body in the morning and at night.
This will help ensure optimal skin quality for your spray tan.

Peak week

7 days before: Exfoliate once a day, apply lotion after exfoliation, apply anti-cellulite cream at night (or morning if you exfoliate at night. Start drinking 1.5 gallons of water a day.
5 days before: Reduce weight in training to about 75% max efforts (you don't want to be sore on stage!)
Shave your entire body, yes if mean everything!
Continue with your lotion, exfoliation, anti-cellulite cream. Continue to drink 1.5 gallons of water.
4 days before
Shave your entire body again
Continue with your lotion, exfoliation, anti-cellulite cream. Continue to drink 1.5 gallons of water.
2 days before
Shave your entire body again
Continue with your lotion, exfoliation, anti-cellulite cream. Continue to drink 1.5 gallons of water.
Get your nails done (you can do this the day before the competition too but make sure you do it well before you get your spray tan).
This will be your final day to workout.
1 days before
Take one final shower and DO NOT shave (this can open your pores and create speckles in your tan.)
Exfoliate but DO NOT moisturize.
Dress in something that can help you stand out for the athletes meeting but pack loose clothes for your spray tan.
Register at the Athlete's Meeting.
Get your first (and maybe second coat of spray tan).
Finish your gallon and a half of water by midnight.

Get some rest! Tomorrow will be a big day!

COMPETITION DAY

Drink only to your thirst.

Do not shower unless the people doing your spray tan told you to.

Get your final coat of spray tan.

Get your hair and make-up done.

Go to athletes meeting.

Put on suit and jewelry.

Get final touches done on your tan and apply glaze (usually spray tan company will do this too).

Rock the stage, girl!

Packing List

This is a comprehensive list so you may not need everything listed. I highly recommend making a copy of this list and making sure you have everything. Inevitably I end up forgetting something at each competition

- A cute robe to wear over your suit on competition day
- Anti-cellulite cream
- Baby wipes- to clean-up
- Bikini
- Bikini Bite and Glaze (if you are not using the tanning service)
- Blow Dryer
- Body Soap
- Brush
- Business Cards
- Cash
- Change of Clothes
- Charger for your iPod, iPad, or phone
- Competition Jewelry
- Competition Make-up
- Competition Shoes
- Copy of competition registration form
- Cotton Balls
- Crazy Glue
- Cute clothes for night show (form fitting dark tank dress)
- Cute outfit for athlete's meeting
- Dark baggy clothes for tanning

Valerie Wiest

- Door mirror (you can get one from target for about $20)
- Exfoliator (scrub or cloth)
- Face Soap
- Fake eye lashes
- Flip Flops
- Hair Clips, hair ties and/or bobby pins
- Hair extensions
- Hair heat protectant
- Hair Spray
- Hair straightener
- Hot rollers
- iPod, iPad, cell phone
- Latex Gloves
- Locking roll along suitcase (carry all of your stuff to the show in this)
- Lotion
- Make-up Brushes
- Make-up Remover
- Mini Sewing Kit
- Mouthwash
- Nail clippers and file
- NPC Card (if you have it or you can buy it at the show)
- Old sheets (if you are staying at a hotel, they may charge if the sheets get stained by your tan)
- Pen or pencil and paper
- Perfume
- Pre measured food and snacks to get you through the day
- Q-Tips
- Regular Make-up

- Resistance Bands (for pumping up)
- Safety pins
- Scissors (you never know when you may need them)
- Self-Tanner (if you are not using the tanning service)
- Sheets (so you don't stain the ones at the hotel)
- Shampoo/Conditioner
- Shine Spray
- Shower Cap (to cover your hair during tanning)
- Stain remover stick
- Supplements
- Tampons
- Teasing comb
- Tooth brush, tooth paste and floss
- Tweezers
- Umbrella
- Volumizing mousse
- Water

Competing with Kids

Many moms want to compete to reclaim their body after the birth of their child. This adds another layer of complication to competing. The mindset for competition tends to be complete sacrifice at all costs to win. However, if you are a mom, you can't sacrifice at the cost of your child. This requires a delicate balance and it should be noted that there will be a tradeoff: you will have less time with your child and you may feel grumpy or tired more often which will affect how you act around your child.

Finding Balance

So how do you find a balance? First, you need to establish boundaries. How far are you willing to go to win a plastic statue? Without demeaning the process of competing, it's important to recognize that some things are just way more important than a bikini competition. Please never sacrifice your child's health or safety to squeeze in your workout, meet your diet or do any of the other steps that are required of you to compete. The bottom line is that it is just not worth it.

Next, you need to make sure that you have everything organized and prepared in advance. From your meal prep and planning to your competition countdown, make sure you schedule everything in and stick to your schedule to the best of your ability. For me, this meant making sure I made batches of grilled chicken and sweet potatoes at the beginning of the week and making sure I packed my cooler the night before. It also meant arranging child care for my competition far in advance and making sure my husband was aware of the competition process.

Finally, don't be too hard on yourself. Competing is hard enough without the added family pressures. If you need to miss one workout or mess up on your diet for one meal, don't let that frustrate or derail you. Just keep doing your best.

Breastfeeding

Breastfeeding is something I really believe in, and when I entered my first bikini competition I was still breastfeeding my son who was 15 months. At the time, I couldn't find much information on this topic and it really stressed me out. Now that I have experienced three competitions while breastfeeding, I can tell you that it is not as big of a deal as I originally thought. Here are the answers to the questions I had:

How will the diet affect my milk supply?

Since I competed for the first time when my son was 15 months, it wasn't a big issue. My supply was well established and he was eating plenty of solids so I didn't have to worry too much about him getting enough milk. That said, I did keep my calories relatively high for a competition diet (around 1800-2000). Breastfeeding burns about 300-500 calories per day and for my normal diet I eat around 2400 calories, so that was enough of a deficit for me to lean down without starving. I was also very well hydrated, drinking over a gallon of water a day. The most important factor in maintaining a healthy supply is breastfeeding regularly. In fact, most lactation consultants will point out that our bodies have adapted to survive through harsh conditions and that women have been able to breastfeed through droughts and famine. That said, I would NOT recommend taking your calories below 1500 for any lactating mama, especially one working out like a fiend. I also would NOT recommend drastically manipulating sodium and water intake in your final week whether or not you are lactating. There have been a few cases recently where competitors have suffered heart and/or pancreas failure due to dehydration.

Can I take supplements?

This is a question you need to ask your doctor. I talked to my doctor and did research on my own before supplementing. The supplements I used were: Protein powder, Glutamine, Calcium/Magnesium/Zinc, Multivitamin, Vitamin E, Collagen, and Biotin. I did NOT use a fat burner. Heck, breastfeeding is its own kind of fat burner, right? Since whey protein is often the main source of protein in baby formula, my doctor said not to worry about protein powder, just make sure there were not a lot of additives or other supplements mixed in. I used Dymatize Elite ISO-100, which has a small ingredient list. It does have Splenda in it though, so if you are not ok with that, you may want to do some research on natural brands of protein powder (Jay Robb, etc.) A great resource for breastfeeding moms is the website Kellymom.com. Here is a link to the page where vitamin supplements are described in relation to breastfeeding: http://kellymom.com/nutrition/vitamins/mom-vitamins/.

Biotin (a B vitamin), calcium, zinc, magnesium, and most of the vitamins in my multivitamin are water soluble and should not affect your breast milk or baby. You need to be careful with your vitamin A & E intake though, since they are fat soluble and can accumulate in your milk. Gultamine and Collagen are both essentially made up of amino acids that occur naturally in the body. Gultamine helps with recovery and Collagen helps maintain healthy skin. Both should not affect your baby if you are taking the recommended dosage. While it is not necessary to take supplements, it is a good idea to supplement vitamins if you are going to be cutting calories while breastfeeding. If you have trouble getting enough protein, you may consider supplementing with a whey shake, especially after your workout when your body is primed to use protein for building muscle.

What about the spray tan?

Closer to the competition, my main concern with breastfeeding was competition day and the tan. Since I had the experience of competing once before I got pregnant, I knew what a pain the spray tan was. It is so easy to mess up your tan and I was really worried that I would not be able to breastfeed and/or hold my baby once I got sprayed. Here's what worked for me: The week before the show I made sure to exfoliate well especially on my chest. I wore "Lily Pads" (silicone nipple covers) to get spray tanned so my baby wouldn't have to eat the tan to breastfeed.

Once tanned and DRY I went home and was able to breastfeed, keeping most of my body covered with a robe or loose henley top. Feeding my son did not really mess up my tan, but I was careful of how much contact he had directly with my skin. I was lucky because two of the shows I participated in were relatively close to my home (less than an hour away). This meant I could feed my son first thing in the morning, drive to the competition site to get hair and make-up, do the pre-judging then come home for a quick break before the night show to feed again. Once I finished the night show I went home to feed him to sleep. I did one competition away from home and I just pumped throughout the day using my Lansinoh electric pump. If you plan on being away from your baby, I recommend pumping at least 3 times during the day. The pump did not mess up my tan or leave lines that were visible outside of my suit.

Photo Shoot

Scheduling a fitness photo shoot to document the hard work that you have put into your body is a great idea. However, doing a photo shoot for the first time can seem a bit intimidating. Here are a few tips to help you to prepare for your first shoot! Also, be sure to check out my interview with top fitness photographer Brian Landis in the Interview section for more tips.

1. Choose a great photographer- This may seem self-explanatory but it really is the key to a successful photo shoot. Remember, you get what you pay for and if you are doing a free photo shoot, expect to work with someone who is not as experienced and just building their portfolio.

Try looking for images you like online or in magazines and find out who did the photographs. Ask around, if a friend is posting gorgeous professional pics on social media ask her who she worked with and how her experience was.

A good photographer will know lighting, help guide you in to poses and make you feel comfortable without pressuring you.

Another point is that if you shoot with a published photographer and they like working with you, they may decide to have your pictures published. This can be a great way to break into fitness modeling!

2. Learn how to pose- It is always a good idea to practice your posing and know what looks good on your body before you do a photo shoot. Also, understand what you want your photos to convey and how to show that. Look online or in magazines for posing ideas and practice them in the mirror at home before the shoot

3. What to bring- Clothes, clothes and more clothes! Bring more than you think you will need, but at least 6-8 looks. Try on your looks before your photo shoot and make sure everything looks good together. New clothes will look best if you can afford it, but at the very least, don't show up in your old dingy sweat stained gear. You will want to bring a few pairs of shoes to go with your looks too. Usually dramatic, more extreme fashion statements are great for photo shoots, but make sure to wear solid colors as busy patterns can distract from your physique. Some photographers work with a stylist and will bring clothes you can wear-- so ask what they recommend. In addition, here is a list of items you may want to bring:

- Baby oil
- Make-up for touch ups- At least a lip gloss, powder and blush.
- Scissors- You never know when they might come in handy
- Snacks- Make sure you have healthy fuel that will make you feel great
- Music- Something fun to help get you in the mood

4. Hair and Make-up: Unless you are really great at doing your own hair or make-up I recommend hiring someone to do it for you. This will ensure that you look your best in your pictures. Bring touch-up make-

up or ask your stylist for a touch-up kit. Ask your photographer who they recommend for hair and make-up if you are not sure where to go. A good photographer will have a great network of professionals to recommend.

5. Body Prep: You want to go into your photo shoot looking great. Think of preparing for your photoshoot just as you would for your competition. This is also the reason many competitors schedule their photoshoot around their competition. A few days after your competition is a great time to book your photo shoot because you will have that left over glow from your spray tan (without the blotchy-ness) and you'll still be in great shape (if you don't go too overboard on your after competition meals). Also, make sure your skin looks great by staying hydrated and applying lotion or baby oil.

How to Get Sponsored

Many people go in to competing with goals of getting sponsored and getting rich. Let me be the one to tell you that it doesn't work that way. Many of the top bikini athletes still have day jobs to supplement the income they make from sponsorships, endorsement deals, modeling etc. While top male bodybuilders earn big bucks in the pro competitions, bikini athletes earn considerably less.

However, having a sponsor can help with all the expenses you incur when you compete, just be mindful of the tradeoff that comes with having a sponsor. Companies that choose to sponsor you are usually looking for a return on their investment so be prepared to "work" for them whether that means spending the day at your sponsor's booth at an event, modeling, or promoting their products on social media. How much time and energy are you willing to dedicate to your sponsorship? You might find that it is more valuable to invest that time and energy into your job and earn more money that way. However, if you are still interested in sponsorship, here are a few tips for getting sponsored:

- Think about what you can offer the company that you would like to sponsor you.
- Giver's Gain: Try to help the company in any way you can before you obtain sponsorship. This could be as simple as writing a blog post about their products or volunteering at their booth at a show. That way, you show the company that you are not just about taking from them but also giving back.
- ASK- I know. I was terrified of getting rejected the first time I requested sponsorship. However, if you don't ask you will never know, the worst the company can say is "no."
- Put together a digital portfolio of information about yourself highlighting what you can do for your sponsors. That way, when you request sponsorship you can show the company exactly

what you have to offer them. This can include statistics on your blog and social media accounts, competitions you have done with your placings, and past or current sponsorships.

The Dark Side of Competing

While bikini competitions can be a fun and positive experience, there is also a dark side that I wanted to make you aware of.

Steroids

The NPC is an untested organization, which means that, although no one should be on steroids or other banned substances, many competitors are. While the bikini look requires the least amount of muscle and the most body fat, you will find that many bikini girls will take steroids and stimulants to help achieve the desired look.

I am not here to judge anyone who decides to take banned substances; however, if you do decide to, I would be very aware of the possible side effects and make sure you are getting them from a trusted source. I also recommend asking your doctor about the substances you plan on taking and getting full blood work before you start anything so that you can see how the drugs are affecting your body.

Full disclosure, I have NEVER taken steroids or other banned substances. Part of my reasoning was because of the possible adverse effects, but part of it was also because I wanted to see what type of progress I could make on my own.

I have also seen many people come off banned substances in a hard way: gaining lots of body fat and/or losing lots of muscle mass.

The main banned substances I have heard of bikini girls taking are clenbuterol (clen), anavar (var) and ephedra (sometimes in an ephedra, caffeine, aspirin stack).

I am not going to go into deep detail about what each of these drugs does; however, I will advise you to be aware that the playing field is not necessarily even for untested competitors. That doesn't mean that a natural athlete can't win, it just means that you have to work that much harder to get to the same level in the same amount of time.

Bikini secrets

Beyond steroids there are a few other (legal) little tricks bikini girls use to get their bikini body. However, that doesn't mean that these secrets aren't controversial.

1. The Squeem: The Squeem is essentially a girdle that some girls use throughout their prep to help reduce the size of their waist. Usually, the Squeem is worn at least 8 hours per day. I can testify to the fact that it works. I lost about an inch and a half from my waist for my first competition. However, the inches come back if you stop wearing the Squeem regularly. Wearing the Squeem for long periods of time can also be very uncomfortable. I also noticed that my back and ab muscles significantly weakened.

Those opposed to the Squeem retort that regular use contorts internal organs in a way that is unhealthy and that the use of such a devise for a competition that is supposed to esteem fitness and health seems counterintuitive

2. Neoprene shorts/clothes- Many coaches suggest wearing neoprene garments during cardio to help sweat out water weight and tighten the appearance of the skin. However, all you will lose is water weight and thus, by drinking you will gain it right back.

3. Cellulite cream- since about 80% of women have cellulite, many use creams to help to reduce its appearance on stage. How much it actually helps is debatable, but some girls swear by it. The kind I have seen most recommended and have actually tried myself is "Beauty Bum transdermal muscle toning lotion" by Beauty Fit. If you have sensitive

skin, be careful with his product as it does make skin red, hot and tingly wherever it is applied.

4. Botox and fillers- If you are over the age of 30, and not blessed with skin as smooth as silk, you may want to consider Botox or other fillers to give you a more youthful appearance. Of course there are risks with injectables so make sure you weigh those against the benefits and choose a knowledgeable, experienced provider if you do decide to use fillers. While I have not used Botox or fillers, many competitors choose to use them. And since "overall physical appearance including complexion, skin tone, poise and overall presentation" is one of the things you will be scored on, it may help your scores, or at least give you that boost of confidence you need to perform better.

5. Breast Augmentation- Almost all the IFBB Bikini Pros have had a breast augmentation, and while I don't recommend getting a breast augmentation just for the sake of competing, the look of full breasts can definitely help balance out the full glutes that are desired in the Bikini Division. However, there are other ways to achieve the look of fullness without getting an augmentation: Stuffing your top and using a molded cup top are two tips for flatter chested girls. Admittedly, I got a breast augmentation about a year after my first competition. It was something I had wanted before competing, since I breastfed my son for two years, but I think I hurried my decision based on the fact that I felt like it was a requirement to do well in competitions. Ultimately though, the breast augmentation didn't really affect my scores and I ended up getting my implants removed about a year and a half later because they affected my chest muscles, were uncomfortable and in my opinion looked disproportionately large on my frame.

Post Competition

Congratulations you competed in your first competition! You placed first and you are on the top of the world! Now you can pig out and eat whatever you want to right??

Valerie Wiest

NO! Don't fall into the trap cycle of binging and starving during competition season. You worked so hard to get your body in the best shape of your life, don't just throw it all away the week after your competition.

I'm not opposed to a treat meal after your competition, but there is no need to go overboard! A nice dessert, a burger with fries, a few slices of pizza, but not all three! It's easy to eat 5,000 calories post competition in a single meal and some people continue that binge for a week or so. Many times a competitor will feel so deprived and entitled at the end of a competition that they will spend the rest of the week binging which can turn into the rest of the month and so on.

Instead, have a small treat and get back on track the next day, slowly increasing your calories. If you have a coach, they can help you come up with a post competition plan. Otherwise, you can slowly add calories back on to your diet (100-300/week) monitoring your weight and making adjustments as necessary.

Not only does this take a huge toll on your body, but it also takes a huge toll on your mental health. The flip flop in weight can cause body image issues which can lead to eating disorders. In addition, competitors may feel pressured to maintain their contest ready physique, which may not be realistic. This can cause depression and feelings of anxiety.

Furthermore, going from goal to lack of goal can be depressing, especially if the contest results were anticlimactic (you didn't place as high as you'd like). You spend so much time, energy and focus on this one goal and once you reach it you may feel lost or without purpose.

There are two ways I have found to help combat these post competition blues. The first remedy is the reverse diet.

The reverse diet is essentially gradually adding calories to your diet to reach a point of stabilization. To do this, add on 100-300 calories per week until you return to your normal diet. This helps your body to regulate the increase of nutrients so that you avoid binging and packing on tons of water weight. It also helps you regulate your sense of hunger.

The next thing I would recommend would be to find a new goal for after the competition. This can be as simple as getting stronger in your lifts or it can be unrelated like learning a new skill. My goal after each competition is usually to get stronger and add muscle mass, but I have also had other goals relating more to my career. These goals help you to reclaim the energy you were focusing on the competition. They also help you stay active and positive, which can help you avoid the blues.

If you do feel like you are suffering from depression, talk to your doctor. Depression is a real problem so don't feel bad or weak if you think you have it. There are many ways medical professionals can help including therapy and medication.

Eating Disorders

Unfortunately, the restrictive dieting and lifestyle of competition can lead to eating disorders or encourage eating disorders in those who are already afflicted. The way we diet and train during a competition is not sustainable. Eating at a caloric deficit for a long time may lead to binges, which often leads to purging in an attempt to control weight. In addition, sometimes competitors feel pressure to stay at their competition weight all year long. However, this may not be possible to maintain in a healthy way. The desire to stay competition ready year round may lead to an unhealthy relationship with food and body image.

Symptoms of eating disorders include:

- Inadequate food intake leading to a weight that is clearly too low.
- Intense fear of weight gain, obsession with weight and persistent behavior to prevent weight gain.
- Self-esteem overly related to body image.
- Frequent episodes of consuming very large amounts of food

- A feeling of being out of control during (the binge) eating episodes.
- Feelings of strong shame or guilt regarding (the binge) eating.
- Eating when not hungry, eating to the point of discomfort, or eating alone because of shame about the behavior.
- Self-induced vomiting.
- Abuse of laxatives

(National Eating Disorders Association, n.d.)

If you feel like your relationship with food and body image has gotten out of control, please don't continue to hide your issues through fitness competitions. I promise, life gets better when you stop obsessing about what and how you eat. Reach out to a trusted friend, family member or medical professional and seek help. You can also call the National Eating Disorder Association helpline at 1800-931-2237. Eating disorders should be taken seriously and can have serious health consequences including death.

Interviews

Fitness Photographer: Brian Landis

About Brian:

Based in Millersville, Maryland, Brian Landis is an internationally published fitness photographer. For several years Brian has pushed his photography skills into the fitness and sports realm. Learning the industry, and gaining years of experience in Maryland shooting a variety of commercial work, paved the way for Brian to make an impact in the fitness industry with his work.

Working with top fitness professionals and amateurs alike gives Brian totally different perspectives and a host of shooting possibilities. His work includes reigning three time Ms Olympia bikini IFBB Pro Ashley Kaltwasser in at least four magazine features. Other top people from the IFBB and the NPC fitness leagues as well as other athletes keep him working all over the country.

Brian is currently a contributing photographer for Inside Fitness Magazine, Inside Fitness Women, Most Fitness and several other fitness related magazines, web sites, etc. His work has been in pretty much every major fitness magazine in the form of a feature, editorial, or advertisement.

What do you think makes a good fitness photographer?

A good fitness photographer is someone who not only has good skills with the camera, but a very good knowledge of lighting. It is impossible to create the type of images that a fitness person will want without understanding the ways of lighting the human form to give it as much three dimensional feel as possible. A fitness background and contacts in the fitness industry are also helpful. Being connected to magazines, companies, etc. will lead to better promotion for the athletes.

How should competitors/fitness models choose a photographer to work with?

I would look at the quality of their work, who they have worked with, the styles they shoot (everyone has at least one style they like to do...some moody, some brighter, some gritty, etc.), their location, then their rates...expect to pay a good photographer for their time.

How much can a competitor/fitness model expect to pay for a shoot?

This is a VERY tough question to answer. Rates from different fitness photographers vary from maybe $300 for a beginning fitness photographer all the way up to $3000.00 for a shoot. It also depends on the length of the shoot and what the images will be used for. Commercial usage is always more expensive than personal usage.

How does a competitor/fitness model's photo get published in a magazine?

There are really only two ways in to a magazine: message the editor of the magazine you want to be in and see if you can get some interest or go through a photographer that contributes to a fitness magazine. Either way you will need some great images to show the editor in the style that magazine likes to use in order to get any interest at all.

What would you suggest a first time fitness model bring to a shoot?

Lots of wardrobe and any props or equipment that will not already be at the location you are going to. Talk to your photographer. If they have no suggestions find a new photographer.

What kinds of outfits photograph well and what gets published?

This depends on what you want to use the images for. Remember "Form Follows Function". If you want to get into a women's fitness magazine you should bring fitness outfits that are stylish and up to date. If you are a woman that wants to get into a men's fitness magazine, then the outfits need to be a little more sexy. The women in them are usually fit but shown in a sexy way (we are talking about male readers here!). Basically, know your audience.

What type of make-up would you suggest? Can a fitness model get away with doing their own make-up?

Women's fitness magazines want clean, natural looking makeup and simple hair styles usually pulled back in a ponytail or braid. For men's magazines or sexier fitness a more glam look for makeup is appropriate but still don't go over the top. DO NOT put on Fake Eye Lashes! Ladies all want to use them, but you don't need them for fitness. Why do you need half-inch long eyelashes to go to the gym? Trust me, you don't need them.

I would suggest using a professional hair and makeup artist if at all possible (and it needs to be a one that knows fitness looks, not fashion). Why hire a great photographer and not look your best? You can do your own, but I don't recommend it to most people especially the inexperienced model.

Would you suggest a competitor go with the show sponsored photographer or find their photographer elsewhere?

This would depend on who the show sponsored photographer is. Like anyone else...they are not all equals. Some are great at shooting stage shots but don't do their own lighting or have connections to magazines, etc. Others do all of that. Choose the best person for what you want to get out of the shoot.

When is the best time to schedule the photo shoot around a competition?

Valerie Wiest

This really depends on you as an individual. Some people are not looking or feeling their best right before or right after the show. If you can stay lean, then a day or two after the competition is great. If you can focus and look great before the competition, I would do that. I like the pre-spray tan look better if possible. I have successfully done both and it really depends on the individual.

How should a competitor prep their body before a shoot (i.e. tan? diet? shaving?)

You have to treat the shoot like a competition. Come in lean and defined for best results. If you are carrying too much water your muscles will not show well. You don't want to be too pale but not fake tan looking either so I would say go with a middle ground on that. Fitness apparel and swimwear (both are often used in fitness images) are typically tight and relatively small in coverage. Be clean shaven for the best appearance.

How much time does a fitness photo shoot usually take?

This depends on what you are shooting but I think 2 hours minimum or 4 hours maximum should get most shoots done right.

Who owns the rights to the photo and are there any restrictions in how the competitor can use the photo?

The photographer always owns the rights to the images they take unless there is a contract that states otherwise. Photographers can decide what the images can be used for on an individual image by image or shoot by shoot basis so make sure you talk to the photographer about the usage. Most photographers will charge more if they will be used commercially. DO NOT give the images to your sponsors or magazines without the approval of the photographer. This will not make anyone happy as there will be an argument at least and a lawsuit at worst. Supplement companies and low end magazine editors are notorious for trying to circumvent paying the photographer by getting images from the model. They know they shouldn't do it but they do it anyway. Do not give them anything. Have them contact the photographer about usage.

How can someone become a paid fitness model?

A big name in the industry or a large social media following will help speed this process up. You need a strong portfolio of images from top photographers to really start getting paid. A good agent could help if you can find one.

What is the biggest mistake you see competitors/fitness models make on their first photo shoot?

They don't treat it like a competition. You should come in lean and fit. You should also think about what you want from the shoot and what you want to do at the shoot for your images. Pose practice in front of a mirror to get comfortable. Facial expressions and body poses are essential. Look at magazines you want to emulate and study them!

Any final advice for fitness competitors/models looking to book a photo shoot?

Be prepared to shoot several times to build a book of work. You will not shoot once then suddenly get paid. You will need a solid portfolio and maybe even some luck to get to being a paid model. Work with the best people you can afford and work hard!

Anything you want to add?

Build that social media following! Instagram, Facebook, Twitter...having a huge following will get you noticed and paid. Look at Michelle Lewin and Paige Hathaway. They make lots of money simply from their social media following.

How can competitors work with you or find out more about you?

Secrets of the Bikini Competitor

Valerie Wiest

If anyone wants to see more of my work it is online at http://www.bfitphoto.com and on IG at @landisphotographic

Most Fitness Magazine Editor: Biani Xavier

About Biani:

Biani Xavier is a nationally ranked bikini body building competitor, sought after lifestyle fitness coach and certified personal trainer based in Potomac, MD – located just outside of Washington, DC. She began a career in modeling at the age of two, in her home country of Brazil, that led to an ongoing and successful career modeling both in the US and abroad. Biani started her fitness career in 2012, after the birth of her second daughter, as a challenge to herself to follow a healthy lifestyle and get back into shape. The result was discovering true joy in caring for her body while pursuing and sharing her tips on fun, healthy eating and exercise with others.

Biani is part owner and Editor in Chief MOST FITNESS Magazine, a monthly, international magazine in both online and print publication. It features celebrities, fashion trends, and in-depth lifestyle stories complimented by extraordinary photographs shot by some of the best photographers from around the globe.

You can find out more about the magazine and subscribe at http://www.mostmagpub.com

How are stories selected for the magazine?

We look at what's trending. Stories are always related to the magazine's main subjects such as fitness, beauty, health and celebrity.

Who typically pitches an article? Is it the fitness model, photographer, columnist or someone else?

All of the above; in addition, we have articles from everyday people who can share their fitness journey, success stories, tips, food recipes, exercise routines and so on. We also reach out to celebrity chefs who can share a tasty, healthy recipe.

Many girls have a dream of being published, what can they do to increase their chances?

It helps to have some kind of following (FB, IG, Twitter, snapchat...) The more people who know them the better. It will ensure the magazine will get the model's followers to look at the magazine and bring in traffic.

Are there any steps they can take to work toward being published?

It's very important to show that you can photograph well since that's a must for magazines. Make sure you have a great photographer who can take good shots of you and make you look like magazine content. Write!! If you can't, have someone do it for you. Pictures could mean nothing without a message, a story, an article to go with it. I think you simply have to do your thing, do it with passion, do it well... The rest will come. People will start noticing you, they will feel inspired by you and eventually the magazines will be interested as well.

What are you looking for in the fitness models you feature in the magazine?

We are looking for stories that sell, it's that simple! Our job is to capture readers' attention and loyalty.

What can a fitness model do to stand out over others?

Do something new, write a book, start a workout routine that will differentiate you from others, and reach out to that magazine. You would be surprised that most magazines would accept your article if it's well put together. They don't know you or know that you have something to share. Reaching out is a must. What do you have to lose?

What is the biggest mistake you see applicants make when trying to get published?

Bad pictures, boring articles, too many grammar errors. Like I said, get awesome pictures done and if you can't write, have someone help you.

Does winning a competition increase the likelihood of a competitor being published?

Yes and no. It depends on what you do after winning. If you win, you have some leverage, so use it wisely. If no sponsors come your way, go after them. It's totally ok to reach out and show that you are interested. Once you land that sponsorship it's easier to also land some fitness modeling and magazine opportunities.

If you lose, don't be discouraged, you can still reach out. If you have the look they are looking for, it may not matter that you weren't placed number 1. They will take a look at you regardless.

Any final advice for an aspiring fitness model?

Be yourself! You will stand out that way. No need to try being someone else. Also, whatever you do, do it with passion. You can't fail!

How can competitors find out more about you and the magazine?

Competitors can go to http://www.mostmagpub.com to view the magazine and subscribe.

NPC & IFBB Competition Judge: Gary Udit

About Gary:

Gary Udit has 30 years of experience as a Personal Trainer. He is the creator of the PERFECT POSING series of instructional DVDs – www.perfectposing.com. He is the promoter of regional, national level NPC events and international IFBB events. He serves as a judge in the NPC and IFBB.

What are you looking for in the ideal bikini physique?

- Balance
- Fit condition
- Not overly muscled

How important is conditioning vs muscle vs stage presence vs beauty?

They all create the Total Package.

What do you recommend for suit choice? How important is bling?

Dark colors work best. Same color bling works well!

What is the most common mistake you see bikini competitors making?

- Too much movement onstage.
- Too much bling

What is one thing (if anything) that bikini girls put too much emphasis on that doesn't really matter to the judges?

They put too much emphasis on moving around in stances and presentation.

Can girls with stretch marks compete and do well? Cellulite?

Someone has to win and someone has to lose so EVERYTHING is looked at, just as hair, nails, makeup.

What do you recommend girls do to prepare for a national competition vs. local competition?

The prep is the same. You always want to be at your best!

What do you recommend for jewelry?

We [the judges] should not remember your accessories. They should simply highlight your look.

How do you recommend girls wear their hair?

Wear your hair DOWN!

Can you give any overall posing tips?

Simply do GREAT stances and hold them for 2 counts.

What is the most common mistake you see girls making in posing?

They move around too much and the judges never really get to see them in a great stance.

Any final advice for competitors?

Be in shape and learn great stances for YOUR body!

How can competitors work with you or find out more about you?

Checkout my website https://garyudit.com/new/posing-seminars/ for Perfect Posing Clinics. They are invaluable!!!

Valerie Wiest

Competition Make-up Artist: Christy Tate

About Cristy:

Cristy Tate is a young entrepreneur. After graduating with a Bachelor's degree in English and a minor in Marketing, she decided to expand on her true passion; makeup. She recently graduated from Paul Mitchell The School Jersey Shore with a licensure in Cosmetology. While attending Paul Mitchell, Cristy was an active member of Design Team, 'Be Nice or Else,' and Phase II, on the clinic floor. Her portfolio includes clients such as Tommie Copper, Reader's Digest and Frye Boots. She plans to continue to work in fashion, media and bodybuilding and touch as many lives as possible.

How long have you been doing hair/makeup for competitors?

I have doing hair and makeup for competitors for about 5 years now. Previously I worked on set for companies such as Tommie Copper, Readers Digest and Frye.

How is doing hair/makeup for competitors different than other types of hair/makeup?

Hair and makeup for shows tends to be more intense. I like to make sure that if my client's hair and makeup is being done at 5am, they will be looking just as fabulous at 8pm after finals!

What brands of makeup do you suggest competitors use?

There are many great brands to invest in, but I recommend trying things out and seeing what works best for your skin type. I also believe that using a primer is necessary when you plan on being dolled up all day. My favorite tend to be Makeup Forever, Kat Von De and MAC, all for different products!

What makeup tools are absolute must haves?

You definitely want a good brush set and a good bronzer or contour kit. These items can help to define your face on the go and give you a much more "put together" look for every day. I also feel that investing some time into maintaining your eyebrows behind the scenes is great to do. If you feel that you are too sensitive to waxing, try threading. This will help you to have a clean space that is outlined well for you or your artist to work with!

What hair products do you suggest competitors use?

Dry shampoo is a MUST!! It is a great way to add volume, cleanliness and a fool-proof way to make your hair last all day. Being a hairdresser as well, I obviously suggest that nothing is "store bought," definitely look into professional products. What is great about the industry I work in is that it is always changing! Within the past year, companies have come out with dry conditioner as well, which can help keep your tresses softer and smoother, but still feel clean.

What hair tools are essential?

I see many competitors using extensions, which I think is a great addition to any style that you may be looking to achieve. Make sure that you are purchasing Remy Human Hair, that way it can be styled and used just as if it is your own. Permanent extensions, that can last 6 months to a year, are also something that competitors can invest in (and I would be more than happy to install them)!

What is the biggest mistake you see competitors making regarding stage makeup?

The biggest mistake I usually see is incomplete makeup looks. Finishing your makeup and making sure that all aspects are complete is extremely important. Competitors also want to avoid being as dark as their body.

Try and compliment the shade of your tan, but also make sure that you keep your face a natural tan, not too dark and not too light!

What is the biggest mistake you see competitors making regarding stage hair?

Stage hair should be complete and have a finished look. Make sure that if you color or lighten your hair, that it is fresh. You put so much hard work and time into your physique and diet and your hair and makeup are just as important. Make sure that whatever style you choose, it is finished, smooth and looks presentable and professional!

What colors do you suggest for the stage make up?

I suggest sticking with colors that are natural to you. Neon shades, bright colors and heavy glitters are not necessarily something I tend to gravitate towards. Glitter can have a negative reflection with all of the lighting and bright colors are something used for a "pop" of color (ie: the lip, a liner, brighter blush).

What style looks best on stage?

Style is really up to the competitor. I make sure to have a thorough consultation with all of my clients and really have an understanding of their personality. The look we are trying to achieve then comes into play, so if you have a vivacious personality, don't hide it!

Should competitors consider changing their hair color?

There is no need to change your hair color unless you would like to. If you plan on doing so, just make sure you are using professional color lines and going to a salon to see a stylist! PS. I am more than happy to assist anyone in that area!

Should competitors use show sponsored makeup/hair artists? Why or why not?

Make sure you chat with the stylist beforehand and are comfortable with their before and after photos, personality and pricing. The day of your show you want to be in good hands. Many show sponsored artists are an excellent way to go, because they are on site and know what to expect with the show.

Should competitors consider learning how to do their own hair/makeup and do you have an good resources for learning?

Learning how to do your own hair and makeup can be an asset in many ways. I personally give private and group lessons, so this can also be a great way to get together with some girlfriends during prep and enjoy yourself! Learning tips, tricks and makeup secrets can help you to dominate on and off stage!

How can competitors find out more about you and how to work with you?

Feel free to check out my website www.cristymtate.com, my Instagram accounts @cristymtate & @belladonnabeauty

I also offer Budoir Packages with a female photographer Bethany, feel free to check her work out:

http://www.bethanybearmorephotography.com/

National Level Competitor: Juana Graves

About Juana:

Juana is a self-proclaimed Military Brat living in Maryland. She has always been physically active and has been involved in sports since middle school. Juana started lifting in 2008 and competing in 2009 and got hooked! In 2016, she was awarded the Overall Bikini Winner at the NPC Philadelphia Classic. Health and fitness are not only Juana's passion but also her lifestyle.

How did you get started in competitions?

I was working out in a gym with various competitors. Out of Curiosity, I got the urge to try it a year later.

What was your first competition like?

Exciting! Definitely a learning experience with no expectations!

What were some lessons you have learned about competing over the years?

1. Your body should fit the required look in the division you want to succeed in.
2. Do research before making a decision! Knowledge is a must in all areas
3. Don't be so hard on yourself. Hard work is supposed to be hard; however, it is rewarding! Patience is a must!

What (if anything) helped most in winning your first overall title?

1. Taking ample time off to fit the requirement of my division! What you do in your off-season will better prepare you for the in-season.
2. Have confidence! All work is worthless unless you show confidence!

Valerie Wiest

Have you competed in any national level shows and if so what was that experience like?

2016 will be my first year. I've been Nationally Qualified 3 times already the past few years, however I felt I was not ready for the National Stage.

Do/Did you use a coach and how was that experience?

From 2013-2015 yes! 2016 I gained expert diet and peak week advice! I also try to learn as much as I can on my own!

What do you suggest a competitor look for in a coach?

Certification, Experience, Desire to Coach, Contest Prep Knowledge, Sincerity

What is your competition diet like?

Proteins, Healthy Fats, Green Veggies, and Carbs

Macros are numbered out depending on my weak and strong areas.

What kind of training program do you follow?

80 percent Lower Body and 20% Upper body and Cardio depending on if I am in or off season.

What exercises can you suggest to help build glutes?

Primaries- Squats, Deadlifts, Hip Thrusts, Lunges

Secondary- Plyometrics, Kickbacks, Isolated Movements

What do you recommend for suit choice? How important is bling?

Jewel Toned Colors - avoid pastel or neon colors

Bling is cool but not overly desired - no disco ball suits, color crystals preferred.

Valerie Wiest

What do you recommend for jewelry?

Chandelier earrings, no hoops or distracting pieces

How do you recommend girls wear their hair?

Down with soft waves or straight but not flat. Avoid up-dos or short hair styles. Extensions are preferred!

Do you do your own hair? make-up? tan?

I go for a professional look or get them professionally done.

Make-up should be complimentary to your skin tone and suit.

What is the hardest part of competing?

Staying sane lol - enjoy the journey and be confident!

What is the most fun/rewarding part of competing?

Meeting all kinds of people from different journeys, sharing the same passion.

Do you stay contest ready all year?

No.... I try to maintain a neutral ground as best as I can but life happens.

Have you felt the effects of post competition depression/binge?

I haven't, I try to regroup with as little stress as possible.

What tips can you give to an aspiring bikini competitors?

Follow through and give it your all! Don't work hard and then present half a package.

Any advice on achieving sponsorship?

Currently my journey, social media and maintaining relationships will definitely help!

How can readers find out more about you?

They can follow me on Instagram @HavanaJuana

Or e-mail me at: CubanBeauty23@gmail.com

Valerie Wiest

My First Competition Re-Cap

I thought it might be helpful to give you a re-cap of my first competition to give you a better idea of what competition day will be like.

The weekend of my competition was a whirlwind. Up until the competition, I was running around like a crazy person trying to get things ready – work, nails, check-in, tanning.

The actual competition day was exciting. I came to my coach's house for her to do my make-up while her friend and amazing hair stylist, Ruth Harper, did my hair. From there, I went to the competition location (only 15 min. away) for the athletes meeting. Once the meeting was over I headed back stage to get another coat of mud (tanner). My tan had gotten really blotchy overnight so I was freaking out about how it would look on stage but the tanning girls assured me no one would be able to tell.

With tan on, I headed back to the hallway (our backstage area) to put on my suit, jewelry and robe and then wait for my turn and wait and wait and wait. There was a lot of waiting. The competition started at 11am but I didn't go on stage until after 1:30pm so I had a lot of time to check out the other competitors. I tried not to psyche myself out or compare myself. About 20 min before It was my turn to go on stage I got my glaze on and Ruth sprayed my hair so that it looked ginormous.

When it was finally my turn to go on stage I was so nervous and excited. The things my coach had said to me in our posing sessions stuck in my head: smile, pretend like you are having the best day of your life. So I did and I got out there and I rocked it. I got into my place on the side stage and was beaming with confidence. Then, my number was called FIRST! I was the first one called for first call outs and they set me up in the middle spot, which usually means you won first place. I was ecstatic!

Valerie Wiest

I could not stop smiling. I strutted off the stage and immediately texted my husband and my coach.

There were a few hours between the pre-judging and the night show (where they hand out awards) so I went home to see my son. Sadly, I think my extreme make-up tan and hair scared him because he would not even come near me. The time went quickly and in what felt like a few minutes, I had to rush back to the competition for another athletes meeting and then…. more waiting. Since most of the judging was done in the morning show, I was not as nervous as I was before but I kept thinking that I would win and worrying about how I would do in the overall.

When the judges lined us up for the night show, we were out of order and there was one girl in front of me. I kept hoping that I would still win and that maybe she was just in front of me for suspense but they ended up calling me as the runner up. I was still ecstatic. My trophy was a sword.

Walking off the stage I was on cloud 9-- finally able to eat what I wanted to, finally able to shower and finally having won! After pictures and congratulations with my coach I went to ask the judges for feedback. It seems the consensus was that I still need to build muscle.

My goal had just been to not place last and I ended up placing second! I was thrilled and officially hooked on competing.

Conclusion

You've made it to the end! Congratulations! I truly wish you success in your competition and hope that you found my book helpful. I am happy to answer any follow up questions that you might have. Just visit my website www.valeriewiest.com/contact. If you found this book helpful, please leave a 5 star review.

Thanks again!

Resources

Suits:

Waterbabies: https://www.waterbabiesbikini.com/

Suits You: http://www.suitsyouswimwear.com/

Ravish Sands: http://www.ravishsands.com/

CJ's Elite: http://cynthia-james.com/

Lydia Conti: http://www.lidiaconti.com/

Tan:

Protan: www.protanusa.com

Liquid Sun Rayz: www.liquidsunrayz.com

Jan Tana: http://jantana.com/

NPC website:

http://npcnewsonline.com/schedules/

My Coach:

Jessica Jessie: www.jessicajessie.com/

Products Mentioned:

http://valeriewiest.com/shop/

Interviewees:

Brian Landis: http://www.bfitphoto.com/

Biani Xavier: http://www.mostmagpub.com/

Secrets of the Bikini Competitor

Valerie Wiest

Gary Udit: https://garyudit.com/new/posing-seminars/

Cristy Tate: http://www.cristymtate.com/

Juana Graves: CubanBeauty23@gmail.com

About the Author

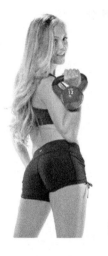

Valerie is a Pilates Instructor, Certified Personal Trainer and Nutritionist, National Level Bikini Competitor and New Mom.

Her passion is sharing health and fitness information with others. Valerie believes that fitness and nutrition are not one size fits all and she strives to educate people on what works for their body. Valerie's hope is that through customized fitness and nutrition people will look better, feel better and get hooked on a healthy lifestyle.

You can find out more about Valerie and sign up to get free tips and information on her website ValerieWiest.com.

Valerie Wiest

Bibliography

Angelo Tremblay, J.-A. S. (1994). Impact of exercise intensity on body fatness and skeletal muscle metabolism. *Metabolism Clinical and Experimental*, 814–818 .

Carol S. Johnston, S. L. (2004). High-Protein, Low-Fat Diets Are Effective for Weight Loss and Favorably Alter Biomarkers in Healthy Adults. *The Journal of Nutrition*, 586-591.

Craig Horswill, P. (n.d.). *The 1.5%-Per-Week Rule Part One: Fat Loss*. Retrieved 11 2, 2014, from KHSAA: http://khsaa.org/sportsmedicine/weight/percentage_part1.pdf

Cribb, P. J. (2006). Effects of Supplement-Timing and Resistance Exercise on Skeletal Muscle Hypertrophy. *Medicine & Science in Sports & Exercise*, 1918-1925.

Crovetti R, P. M. (1998). The influence of thermic effect of food on satiety. *European Journal of Clinical Nutrition* , 482-488.

Earle, T. R. (2008). *Essentials of Strength Training and Conditioning - 3rd Edition*. Chicago: Human Kinetics Publishers.

Gerson E. Campos, T. J. (2002). Muscular adaptations in response to three different resistance-training regimens: specificity of repetition maximum training zones. *European Journal of Applied Physiology*, 50-60.

Hamid R Farshchi, M. A. (2005). Beneficial metabolic effects of regular meal frequency on dietary thermogenesis, insulin sensitivity, and fasting lipid profiles in healthy obese women. *American Journal of Clinical Nutrition*, 16-24.

Heather J. Leidy, N. S. (2007). Higher Protein Intake Preserves Lean Mass and Satiety with Weight Loss in Pre-obese and Obese Women. *Obesity: A research journal*, 421-429.

Institute of Medicine of the National Academies. (2005). *Dietary Reference Intakes for Energy, Carbohydrate, Fat, Fatty Acids, Cholesterol, Protein and Amino Acids.* Washington: National Academies Press.

JS Volek, N. D. (1999). Performance and muscle fiber adaptations to creatine supplementation and heavy resistance training. *Medicine & Science in Sports & Exercise* , 1147-156.

Kraemer WJ, A. K.-M. (2002). American College of Sports Medicine position stand. Progression models in resistance training for healthy adults. *Medicine and Science in Sports and Exercise*, 364-380.

National Eating Disorders Association. (n.d.). *Types & Symptoms of Eating Disorders*. Retrieved April 18, 2015, from National Eating Disorder Association: http://www.nationaleatingdisorders.org/types-symptoms-eating-disorders

NPC BIKINI DIVISION RULES. (n.d.). Retrieved April 12, 2015, from NPC News Online: http://npcnewsonline.com/npc-bikini-division-rules/